INCONTINENCE AND ITS MANAGEMENT

Second Edition

INCONTINENCE AND ITS MANAGEMENT

SECOND EDITION

Edited by DOROTHY MANDELSTAM

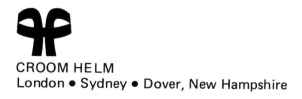

CROOM HELM
London ● Sydney ● Dover, New Hampshire

© 1980 Dorothy Mandelstam
Second Edition © 1986 Dorothy Mandelstam
Croom Helm Ltd, Provident House, Burrell Row,
Beckenham, Kent BR3 1AT
Croom Helm Australia Pty Ltd, Suite 4, 6th Floor,
64-76 Kippax Street, Surry Hills, NSW 2010 Australia

British Library Cataloguing in Publication Data

Incontinence and its management. —2nd ed.
   1. Faeces—Incontinence 2. Urine—
Incontinence
   I. Mandelstam, Dorothy
   616.6'3   RC921.I5
   ISBN 0-7099-3580-3

Croom Helm, 51 Washington Street,
Dover, New Hampshire 03820, USA

Library of Congress Cataloging in Publication Data
Main entry under title:

Incontinence and its management.

   Bibliography: p.
   Includes index.
   1. Urine—incontinence. 2. Feces—incontinence.
I. Mandelstam, Dorothy.
RC921.15148   1986   616.8'49   85-27001
ISBN 0-7099-3580-3 (Pbk.)

IBM Typeset by Words & Pictures Ltd (formerly Elephant Productions)
Thornton Heath, Surrey

Printed and bound in Great Britain by
Biddles Ltd, Guildford and King's Lynn

CONTENTS

FOREWORD

This book must be welcomed as a definitive account of the symptom of incontinence in adults. It is an attempt to gather together the many aspects of a distressing and often crippling condition which affects individuals of all ages but is of particular significance in the old. It may make normal life impossible, may cause embarrassment to friends and relatives however well-meaning who tend to regard it with disgust. Indeed this attitude goes back to the nursery and to all our childhoods when our infantile failures were a source of shame and often of punishment.

The book's origin lies in the work of Dorothy Mandelstam of the Disabled Living Foundation and Royal Free Hospital where so much is done for those unfortunate enough to suffer disability of one kind or another, often not through their own fault.

A distinguished and authoritative team of authors has been assembled to write about the mechanisms and management of incontinence in all its aspects. The team includes urologists, surgeons, physicians, geriatricians, gynaecologists, a general practitioner, nurses, community physicians, a physiotherapist, a psychologist and a social worker.

We each in our own special field tend to become preoccupied with our own clinical problems and the solutions we hope to offer. But this book shows that incontinence is often a complex symptom requiring careful teamwork and the co-operation of more than one discipline in the medical and paramedical field.

To have brought together such a diverse team of authors and to have welded them into a comprehensive book and one written with such understanding is an unparalleled achievement.

Dame Josephine Barnes

MA, DSc(Hon), DM, MD(Hon), FRCP, FRCPI (Hon), FRCS, FRCOG.
Consulting Obstetrician and Gynaecologist,
Charing Cross Hospital and Elizabeth
Garrett Anderson Hospital.
President, British Medical Association, 1979-80.

PREFACE

This book is about incontinence in adults. It is intended primarily for doctors, nurses and members of the paramedical professions. By including a glossary of technical terms, it is hoped that the scope of the book will include the more adventurous non-medical reader and thus be of value to patients, relatives and others who may have experienced or witnessed the demoralising effect of the problem.

There is inevitable overlapping, as the various contributors approach the same subject from different professional standpoints. The main aim of the book is to make the point that with modern methods of treatment, and a modicum of patience, incontinence is not necessarily an irreversible condition. In many cases it can be cured altogether, and in others it can be alleviated to an extent which results in the rehabilitation of the patient and the restoration of his dignity and self-respect.

Finally the book ought to be of interest to administrators and planners such as those in the Department of Health and Social Security. A significant part of the funds and resources available to them are at present expended in nursing patients who have been institutionalised solely or mainly because they have been classified as incontinent. For purely demographic reasons this group will in the coming years consume a progressively larger proportion of these resources. For a relatively modest outlay diverted to education, training and publicity it should be possible to impart to doctors, nurses and other staff in the health and social services knowledge of the techniques and facilities that will rehabilitate many of these patients. With the results of the surveys reported in Chapter 14, it should be possible to estimate, at least roughly, the size of the problem, the cost of the service at present provided, and the magnitude of the saving that could be achieved. These financial resources could then be diverted from institutional care to the improvement of domicilary services, particularly in respect of the training of staff. With this increase in understanding and skill, and the provision of realistic additional support, home care for patients would be not only preferable, but also possible.

ACKNOWLEDGEMENTS

I would like to thank Dr Monnica Stewart for her encouragement and support, and Dr M. Gray for her advice. My thanks are also due to Mrs Margaret Gillson for all her assistance, to my mother Dorothy Hillier for her help in the preparation of the final manuscript and to Professor Joel Mandelstam for his editorial criticism.

Acknowledgment is also made to Lady Hamilton, Chairman of the Disabled Living Foundation, as she was one of the first to focus attention on the personal consequences of incontinence.

Dorothy Mandelstam

INTRODUCTION

Incontinence is a devastating symptom with personal and social consequences often far more distressing than the root cause, which may be comparatively simple. For diverse reasons it has received little recognition and understanding from either doctors or nurses. The subject does not receive sufficient consideration in the training of the health professionals and consumer demand is restricted because of the embarrassment and shame which is associated with the symptom and lack of knowledge on the part of the patient of what can be achieved by treatment.

There has been scant study of this particular symptom although in the last two decades medical interest and research have been steadily increasing. The International Continence Society provides a forum for such work and the first epidemiological survey in the UK of the incidence of both urinary and faecal incontinence in the community is in progress (see Chapter 14).

All the contributors to this book recognise the general problems and add to the understanding of incontinence in their own particular fields. By bringing their expertise between the covers of one book it is hoped to add to the overall comprehension of the subject.

It becomes clear that in addition to causative organic factors, emotional and situational ones have to be considered. There is an emphasis on the problems in older age groups; this is not surprising as the average age of the population is increasing, and this is reflected in hospitals and residential homes.

All contributors have stressed that the search for the aetiology of the symptom is of paramount importance, but the depth of investigation must vary. Unfortunately, the initial assessment which needs to be made by members of the primary health care team or by specialists is often omitted. As the general physician concludes: 'If the patient and the relatives are to be spared the tribulations which are attendant on incontinence, it behoves physicians to make an accurate assessment of its cause as a first step towards its prevention or cure.'

The initial chapters (1-4) are a summary of our existing knowledge, with definitions of some new physiological concepts and techniques of investigation following upon research and clinical work in specialised units. The urologist has outlined in some detail the basic physiology of micturition (Chapter 1). Investigation and treatment are dealt with by both urologist and gynaecologist who, while covering similar ground, complement each other (Chapters 2 and 3). New aspects of pelvic floor physiology are to be found in the contributions of the urologist and the general surgeon (Chapters 1 and 4) and the latter in his chapter on faecal incontinence emphasises the importance of prevention by minimising all forms of trauma to the pelvic floor muscles. The gynaecologist writing on re-education of the muscles of the pelvic floor endorses the view that the need for restoration of pelvic floor functions by non-surgical measures is still insufficiently appreciated (Chapter 10).

The importance of the sufferer's own attitude, as well as that of the attendant, is emphasised by several of the authors. The interaction of the two is particularly relevant to the successful management of incontinence especially if any form of institutional care is needed. The understanding of these dynamics in training is stressed by the nurse, clinical psychologist and social worker (Chapters 11, 12 and 13). If individual needs are taken into account in management there will be far less work of a routine and unpleasant nature for the attendant.

The need to look at environmental factors is obvious and often provides a simple cure to incontinence. The provision of a suitable receptacle in hospital when the patient needs it is an example, although such simple measures are often overlooked. The general practitioner's assessment during a joint visit with the district nurse enables them together to advise in the home (Chapter 8). Housing alterations can sometimes provide an answer, and knowledge of environmental resources is emphasised by the community physician (Chapter 7).

Still many problems remain. Free discussion of the subject would lessen the taboo and so encourage self-help and the seeking of professional advice. Publicity of the subject through the media is difficult to achieve, and more explicit information from the health and social services is needed. There appear to be barriers to both.

In-service training is an immediate requirement and the development of a Nurse Incontinence Adviser in each health district would be a great advance in this respect (see Chapter 9). Her teaching role could have a real impact on patient care as well as on staff morale, as both are poor when the problem is not understood. Furthermore, as the physician in geriatric medicine comments (Chapter 6A), without such education and accompanying change of attitude staff levels will continue to fall, as nurses opt out from what appears to be an intolerable situation. The distribution of expertise and material resources throughout the country varies widely. Future development will depend on an increasing number of professionals who, like the contributors to this book, are concerned about incontinence and its consequences.

INTRODUCTION TO THE SECOND EDITION

Six years have elapsed between the first and second edition of this book. Services to the incontinent patient have increased but are still far from widespread.

Sadly one of the contributors — Sir Alan Parks — has died prematurely. Fortunately others have continued with his research into sphincter innervation of the pelvic floor.[1]

A professional group including a number of the contributors to this book, published a report 'Action on Incontinence'[2] in 1983, reviewing the whole subject of incontinence. Its findings revealed a failure of professional education at all levels. However, the subject of gynaecological urology is now a recognised medical speciality, and the first post-basic course for nurses in the 'Promotion of Continence and Management of Incontinence' has been approved.[3] The developing role of the nurse has necessitated revision of Chapter 9 for this new edition.

The prevalence surveys carried out during the last few years at the Epidemiology and Medical Care Unit at Northwich Park Hospital have now been completed and the details as well as the implications are included as a new chapter (14). There is also a further chapter on medical practice in incontinent geriatric patients (Chapter 6B). Other chapters remain exactly as in the first edition.

Notes

1. Snooks, S.J., Setchell, M., Swash, M., Henry M.M. (1985), 'Injury to Innervation of Pelvic Floor Sphincter Musculature in Childbirth', *Lancet*, 8 Sept., 546-50.
2. King's Fund (1983), 'Action on Incontinence', King's Fund Project Paper, no. 43.
3. English National Board (1984), 'An Introduction to Promotion of Continence and Management of Incontinence', Course 978, post-basic clinical studies.

1 NORMAL MICTURITION AND ITS CONTROL

Roger C.L. Feneley

Micturition does not conform to a uniform pattern, but exhibits a wide variation from infancy to old age and between one individual and the next. What is normal to one may be abnormal to another. The difference between normal and abnormal function is dependent on its voluntary control and the many factors which influence this are still not fully understood. Loss of this control leads to urinary incontinence and a potential problem that requires no emphasis.

Modern medical technology has provided new methods of investigating disorders of the urinary tract. These have placed emphasis on the study of bladder and urethral function rather than their anatomical appearance. During the past twenty years physiological measurement using urodynamic techniques has passed rapidly from the field of academic research to its present position as a service commitment on which clinical management can both be based and monitored. The formation of the International Continence Society in 1971 witnessed the wide growth of interest developed in the study of continence, stimulating the challenge of treating incontinence and amending many classic concepts.

The Micturition Cycle

Normal micturition involves the ability to store and to void urine at will in suitable places and at convenient times, and thus it constitutes not a single act but a cycle of events. This cycle can vary, so that at one extreme there is an individual with the 'camel' bladder that empties twice a day, whilst at the other there is one who voids every two hours by day and even accepts disturbance to void at night as normal. In mechanical terms the bladder may be compared to a reservoir during storage and a pump during voiding and the urethra provides the necessary resistance, not only to sustain continence but also to allow complete evacuation. In dynamic terms continence is maintained, so long as the pressure within the bladder is lower than the urethral resistance and urine escapes when this balance is reversed. This synergetic relationship between bladder and urethra depends both on its anatomical structure and its physiological control.

The Bladder

The detrusor muscle forms the smooth muscle of the fundus of the bladder and it consists of a meshwork of interlacing bundles, not clearly defined into layers, mounted upon the base or trigone of the bladder. Donker *et al.*[1] were unable to find any evidence to show continuity between the detrusor and the urethral smooth muscle. During the storage phase of micturition this muscle accommodates to an increasing volume of urine and this physical characteristic has been termed compliance. Compliance indicates the relationship between the change in volume and pressure during filling.

During normal filling the compliance approximates infinity until the limit of distensibility of the bladder is reached. Any factor such as inflammation or fibrosis that affects this property of the smooth muscle thus influences the compliance or capacity of the bladder. On voiding, the contraction of the interwoven muscle bundles causes a reduction in all the dimensions of the bladder and thus facilitates complete evacuation of the viscus.

The trigone provides the firm base of the bladder and includes both the ureteric and the internal urethral orifices. There are two distinct muscular layers. The superficial trigonal muscle is in continuity with the longitudinal layer of the ureteric muscle cranially and it extends into the proximal urethra distally. The deep trigonal muscle affords the attachment for the detrusor muscle and Gosling[2] has suggested that this layer should be termed the trigonal detrusor muscle.

Hutch[3] emphasised the importance of the flat base-plate of the trigone in the maintenance of continence and his radiological studies showed that this flat plate was transformed into an open funnel leading into the urethra during voiding. Jeffcoate and Roberts[4] used radiological methods to delineate the angle between the bladder base and urethra. They suggested that the loss of the posterior urethro-vesical angle with funnelling of the junction at rest and increased downward movement to the bladder base on straining could be associated with incontinence due to urethral sphincter dysfunction.

The Urethra

The sphincteric mechanisms of the urethra are extremely complex and there is a basic difference between male and female anatomy. The essential components lie between the internal urethral meatus and the external urethral sphincter and they consist of elastic tissue, detrusor muscle, and urethral smooth and striated muscle, as well as the contribution from the skeletal muscle of the pelvic floor.

Adequate compression of the mucosal folds of the urethra provides the necessary watertight closure for maintaining continence and this must be sufficient to resist any increase in intra-abdominal pressure transmitted to the bladder during urine storage. The mucosal lining consists of folds of transitional cell epithelium in the male, but stratified squamous epithelium is present in the lower third of the female urethra. This is under the hormonal influence of oestrogen and thus may show changes related to this particularly in the post-menopausal woman.[5]

The terminology previously used to describe the internal sphincter and external sphincter raises semantic discussion and to overcome this the terms proximal urethral or bladder neck sphincter mechanism and the distal urethral mechanism have been suggested.[6] The proximal urethral mechanism includes the concentration of elastic tissue in this region, together with the loops of detrusor muscle that sweep around the internal meatus and the urethral smooth muscle itself. Gosling has described a distinct circular smooth muscle or pre-prostatic sphincter in the male in this region, which is richly supplied by sympathetic nerves, and this appears to be involved in the mechanism of ejaculation, preventing retrograde flow of seminal fluid into the bladder (see Figure 1.1). In the female, no sphincter is present, but the smooth muscle runs mainly in a longitudinal or oblique direction.

Gosling's work with the electron microscope and histochemical techniques have also clarified the detailed anatomy of the striated external urethral sphincter. This was previously considered to be a peri-urethral muscle, but Gosling has shown that it is an intrinsic muscle of the urethra. In the male it surrounds the urethra, distal to the verumontanum of the prostate and it is quite separate from the striated musculature of the pelvic floor. In the female, this intrinsic striated musculature is most prominent in the middle-third of the urethra which it surrounds, but it extends both proximally and distally, thus exerting its influence on the whole length of the urethra (see Figure 1.2).

Gosling's studies have also demonstrated that this intramural striated muscle is innervated by autonomic nerves from the parasympathetic supply rather than the pudendal nerve as previously considered. The muscle is classified as a 'slow twitch' type, capable of sustained contraction over long periods of time.

Figure 1.1: The Male Lower Urinary Tract: A. Midline Sagittal Section B. Coronal Section

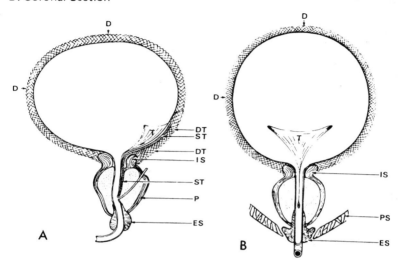

Key: D, detrusor muscle; DT, deep trigonal muscle; T, trigone; ST, superficial trigonal muscle; IS, internal urethral or pre-prostatic sphincter; P, prostatic capsule; ES, external urethral sphincter; PS, peri-urethral striated muscle of pelvic floor. Source: Reproduced by kind permission of Professor J.A. Gosling.

The peri-urethral skeletal musculature of the pelvic floor lies outside the urethra and this is supplied by the pudendal nerve. Functionally, this is of the 'fast twitch' type and is capable of rapid contraction over short periods of time. This provides the explanation for the voluntary contraction, which can stop micturition, and the reflex mechanism of contraction that occurs on sudden coughing or straining. Muscle spindles are present in this pelvic floor muscle and these respond to any changes in tension arising from increased intra-abdominal pressure (see Chapter 4, p. 84). Pudendal nerve block does not relax the external urethral sphincter and the reason for this was not previously appreciated.

The prostate gland in the male occupies that part of the urethra between the proximal and the distal sphincter mechanisms. Enlargement of the gland not only lengthens the urethra but can cause compression

Figure 1.2: Coronal Section of Female Lower Urinary Tract

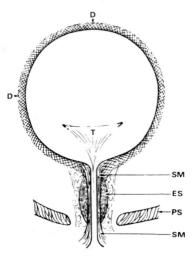

Key: D, detrusor muscle; T, trigone; SM, smooth muscle of urethra; ES, external urethral sphincter; PS, peri-urethral striated muscle of pelvic floor.
Source: Reproduced by kind permission of Professor J.A. Gosling.

of this region and in addition it may compromise the proximal urethral mechanism. Prostatectomy ablates the proximal urethral mechanism, but continence is maintained so long as the distal sphincter remains intact. In cases where the distal urethral mechanism is injured, such as those associated with fractures of the pelvis, continence can be maintained if the proximal urethral mechanism is undamaged. Thus, in practical terms continence requires in both males and females either an intact proximal or distal sphincter mechanism and if both are deficient, incontinence results.

The Neurological Control

The delicate balance between the detrusor and the sphincter mechanisms is maintained by the co-ordinated reflex activity of the autonomic and somatic nerves. These are mediated peripherally by the afferent and efferent pathways between the lower urinary tract and the micturition centre in the second, third and fourth sacral segments of the spinal cord, and centrally by the modulating inhibitory and facilitatory influence of the higher centres in the nervous system.

The parasympathetic nerves arise from the sacral cord as pre-ganglionic axons and, after relaying in the pelvic ganglia, their short postganglionic fibres supply the detrusor, the smooth muscle of the urethra and the intramural striated muscle of the external sphincter. The parasympathetic component stimulates detrusor contraction via its cholinergic nerve endings, which are uniformly distributed throughout the muscle. The parasympathetic nerves to the urethral sphincter zone maintain the urethral closure and, if these nerves are damaged during extensive pelvic surgery or as a result of diabetic neuropathy, the urethral closing mechanisms may be affected.

The pudendal nerves arise from the same segments of the spinal cord and these supply the striated musculature of the pelvic floor. Afferent nerves carried in both the parasympathetic and pudendal pathways convey proprioceptive and exteroceptive sensory impulses from the bladder, urethra and pelvic floor. These provide not only sensory awareness to the cerebral cortex but are an integral part of the feedback mechanisms in the spinal cord. Thus an increase in intra-abdominal pressure, with afferent stimulation from the muscle spindles in the pelvic floor and the abdominal cavity, results in reflex contraction of the pelvic floor. Bladder filling also causes afferent discharge, which stimulates pelvic floor contraction, and this contraction not only supports and compresses the urethra, but also potentiates inhibition of detrusor contraction.

The role of the sympathetic nerves from the thoraco-lumbar outflow (D11-L1) has received particular interest as a result of the detailed anatomical and neuropharmacological studies in recent years. It has been shown that the distribution of the alpha-adrenergic receptors at their nerve terminals are mainly distributed in the smooth muscle of the proximal urethra, whereas the beta receptors are in the fundus of the bladder. The alpha receptors respond to noradrenaline release by stimulating contraction, whereas the beta receptors relax smooth muscle. Evidence is also available that the sympathetic nerves synapse on the pelvic ganglia, blocking parasympathetic transmission and, by these mechanisms, sympathetic nervous activity promotes urine storage. Despite progress, the understanding of the role of the autonomic mechanisms in the control of micturition is far from complete. Retrograde ejaculation is known to occur following lumbar sympathectomy, but no clinical effect on urinary continence is apparent.

The Central Control of Micturition

The afferent impulses from the lower urinary tract pass up to the brain in the posterior columns and the lateral spinothalamic tracts, relaying at all levels between the sacral cord and the cerebral cortex, particularly in the medulla and the thalamus. The cortical centres are situated in the region of the anteromedial aspect of the frontal lobe, the anterior cingulate gyrus and the paracentral lobule. Bladder sensation of fullness and voiding is represented bilaterally in the spinal thalamic tracts, so that normal bladder awareness is only lost if both tracts are divided.

Any disturbance of the central nervous system may cause disorders of micturition, but the details of the pathways and the mechanisms involved with this control are sparse. Studies of pathological lesions caused by brain injuries, tumours, leucotomies and cerebrovascular problems[7] and the original experimental studies in cats[8] have provided some details. Lesions affecting the frontal lobe can alter the pattern of micturition, increasing or decreasing the frequency of micturition or affecting the social awareness of incontinence. The paracentral lobule controls the activity of skeletal musculature, so that lesions in this area may induce retention of urine by causing sustained pelvic and perineal muscular contraction. The hypothalamic area is the major centre controlling autonomic function. The higher centres suppress detrusor contractions and the main influence of the brain is to inhibit micturition. The corticofugal pathways to the sacral cord pass via the corticospinal and reticulospinal tracts to the sacral micturition centre.

Practical Aspects of Lower Urinary Tract Function

Urodynamic, radiological and electromyographic studies have introduced methods of assessing micturition, which have direct clinical application. This account is not intended to provide details of the techniques, but rather to present the type of information that can be obtained (see Figures 1.3 to 1.9).

Figure 1.3: Sphincterometry — Diagram Illustrating the Withdrawal of the Profile Catheter from the Bladder, and the Site of the Maximum Urethral Pressure at the External Urethral Sphincter.

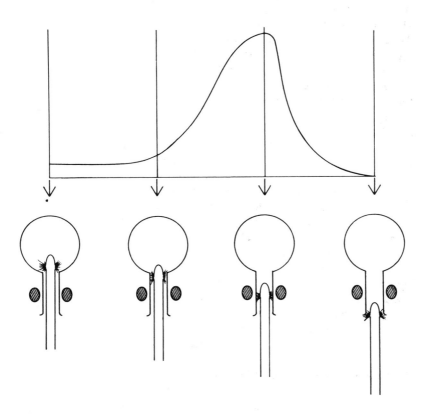

Figure 1.4: Equipment for Recording the Filling and Voiding Cysto-metrogram

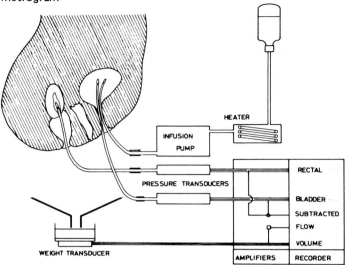

Figure 1.5: A Normal Report

REPORT OF URODYNAMIC INVESTIGATION

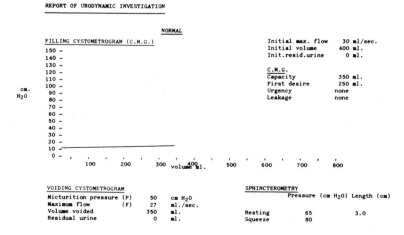

Note: The maximum urine flow rates are measured twice: first when the patient arrives for investigation (Initial Max Flow) and then at the time of the voiding cystometrogram. The initial volume of urine passed was 400 ml and the cystometric capacity of the bladder was 350 ml. The micturition or detrusor pressure on voiding was within the normal range. Sphincterometry showed a normal maximum urethral closure pressure and voluntary contraction of the distal urethral sphincter on being asked to 'squeeze'.

Figure 1.6: A Hypersensitive Bladder   *Sensory Urgency*

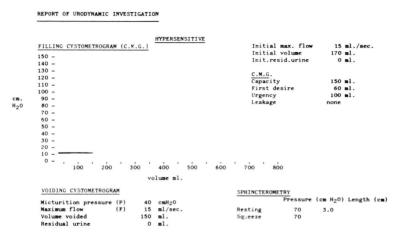

REPORT OF URODYNAMIC INVESTIGATION

HYPERSENSITIVE

FILLING CYSTOMETROGRAM (C.M.G.)

Initial max. flow	15 ml./sec.
Initial volume	170 ml.
Init.resid.urine	0 ml.

C.M.G.

Capacity	150 ml.
First desire	60 ml.
Urgency	100 ml.
Leakage	none

VOIDING CYSTOMETROGRAM

Micturition pressure (P)	40	cmH2O
Maximum flow	(F)	15	ml/sec.
Volume voided		150	ml.
Residual urine		0	ml.

SPHINCTEROMETRY

	Pressure (cm H2O)	Length (cm)
Resting	70	3.0
Squeeze	70	

Note: The functional bladder capacity is reduced and urgency of micturition was noted in filling to 100 ml.

Figure 1.7: A Hypotonic Bladder

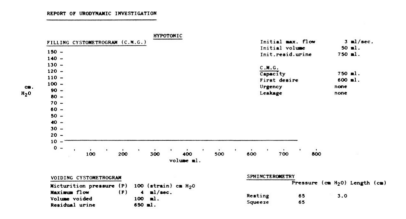

REPORT OF URODYNAMIC INVESTIGATION

HYPOTONIC

FILLING CYSTOMETROGRAM (C.M.G.)

Initial max. flow	3 ml/sec.
Initial volume	50 ml.
Init.resid.urine	750 ml.

C.M.G.

Capacity	750 ml.
First desire	600 ml.
Urgency	none
Leakage	none

VOIDING CYSTOMETROGRAM

Micturition pressure (P)	100 (strain)	cm H2O
Maximum flow	(F)	4	ml/sec.
Volume voided		100	ml.
Residual urine		650	ml.

SPHINCTEROMETRY

	Pressure (cm H2O)	Length (cm)
Resting	65	3.0
Squeeze	65	

Note: A large capacity bladder. Bladder sensation was reduced and the first desire to micturate was noted on filling to 600 ml. Maximum urine flow rates were very low and micturition or detrusor pressure was related to abdominal straining.

Figure 1.8: An Unstable Bladder

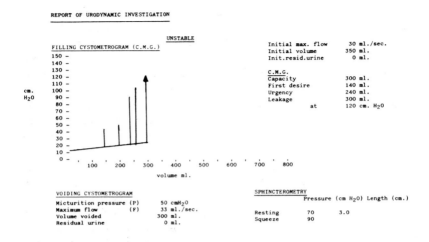

Note: Normal maximum urine flow rates. Detrusor contractions above 15 cm H$_2$O occured on the filling cystometrogram. These patients often show well-developed voluntary contraction of the distal urethral sphincter.

Figure 1.9: An Obstructed Bladder

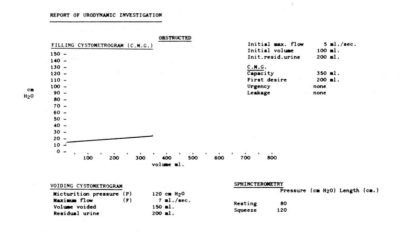

Note: Reduced maximum urine flow rates. A raised micturition or detrusor pressure on voiding of 120 cm H$_2$O.

The Urethral Pressures

Measurement of the urethral pressure can give a useful guide to the relative contributions of the sphincteric mechanisms. Various techniques are used employing fluid- or gas-filled catheters or microtip transducers. The perfusion method described by Brown and Wickham[9] is commonly employed, recording the urethral pressure profile. A fine profile catheter, which has two small side openings, is set about 5 cm from its tip and is perfused with saline solution at a rate of 2 ml/min. This catheter is withdrawn from the bladder through the sphincteric zone of the urethra. The pressure in the catheter is recorded by means of a strain gauge transducer and the profile measures the resistance of the urethral walls opposing the escape of the perfusing fluid from the side openings of the catheter. The profile is graphically displayed and the site of the maximum urethral pressure is usually situated at the level of the external urethral sphincter. If the patient is asked to contract the pelvic floor during the investigation, an indication of the voluntary ability to contract these muscles can be achieved. By subtracting the bladder pressure from the maximum urethral pressure, the maximum urethral closure pressure is noted.

Abrams[10] has described the use of sphincterometry in patients with prostatic obstruction and has pointed out its value, both in those who present borderline indications for operative treatment or those who develop incontinence following prostatic surgery.

The maximum urethral closure pressure in pre-menopausal women is 50-75 cm H_2O, and 40-50 cm H_2O in the post-menopausal state. Men under 45 yrs have pressures of 60-90 cm H_2O and over 45 yrs 60-80 cm H_2O. In women with incontinence, the maximum urethral pressure is usually reduced. Enhorning[11] emphasised that intra-abdominal pressure is transmitted to the proximal urethra, thus providing a passive mechanism of closure. Loss of this transmission of pressure to the urethra may be associated with stress incontinence.

Cystometry

The measurement of bladder pressure during filling and voiding gives a dynamic record of detrusor function. The investigation is of necessity invasive, requiring one catheter to fill the bladder and another to record the pressure within it. Since changes of abdominal pressure are transmitted to the bladder, simultaneous recording of rectal pressure is undertaken and, by electronic subtraction of this from the total bladder pressure, the intrinsic detrusor pressure is derived.

The Filling Cystometrogram

During the filling phase, the detrusor pressure normally remains below 15 cm H_2O until voiding is performed. The first desire to micturate is usually experienced at a volume of 150-200 ml and the bladder capacity is noted when sensation of fullness is experienced at about 350-500 ml.

The filling cystometrogram thus gives information regarding bladder sensation, which may be referred either to the abdomen or perineum and the sensory awareness of the bladder may be increased or decreased. The maximum cystometric capacity can also be measured. In a normal subject there is no evidence of detrusor contraction during filling and inhibition of contraction of the detrusor continues until voiding is established. A bladder which is shown objectively to contract spontaneously or on provocation when the patient is attempting to inhibit micturition, is termed unstable (see Figure 1.8).[12] The unstable bladder is a feature of young children and young adults with diurnal-nocturnal enuresis. About ten per cent of the population have been estimated to retain unstable bladders throughout their life, but the condition may arise in pathological states, such as a secondary phenomenon to obstructive uropathy or related neurological abnormalities, when the term uninhibited bladder is commonly applied.

The Voiding Cystometrogram

The measurement of bladder pressure during voiding is combined with simultaneous recording of the urine flow rates. The measurement of urine flow has become a simple and practical investigation with the introduction of the weight transducer[13] that measured both urine volume and, by differentiation, the flow rate. A variety of differing methods are now available. Interpretation of flow rates for volumes of less than 200 ml on voiding can be misleading and should not be considered representative. The normal flow shows a rapid increase, reaching a maximum within one-third of the total voiding time and the maximum flow rate is taken as the representative value.

These values vary with age and sex and the following measurements are estimates of the lower limit of the normal range:[14]

Males under 40	22 ml/sec
Males 40-60	18 ml/sec
Males over 60	13 ml/sec
Females under 50	25 ml/sec
Females over 50	18 ml/sec

The detrusor pressure recorded during voiding normally rises to about 40-60 cm H_2O in men and 30-50 cm H_2O in women. A poor urine flow rate may be the result of a weak detrusor contraction, in which case the detrusor pressure is low, or it may be related to obstruction in the outflow tract, when detrusor pressures of 100 cm or more may be recorded. When bladder emptying is associated with irregular detrusor contractions or assisted by abdominal straining, an interrupted flow pattern may be demonstrated. Some women achieve rapid bladder emptying with only a marginal increase in detrusor pressure.

Considerable debate has centred on the triggering mechanism that initiates voiding. Muellner[15] considered that it was started by relaxation of the pelvic floor, whereas Hinman *et al.*[16] postulated that it was related to contraction of the detrusor. Tanagho *et al.*[17] using a specially designed catheter for measuring urethral pressures, demonstrated a drop in the urethral pressure a few seconds before voiding, so that urethral pressure and detrusor pressure equilibrated before detrusor contraction commenced.

With the introduction of the image intensifier, cine-radiology of the lower urinary tract during voiding could be undertaken, thus avoiding exposure of the patient to high radiation effects. Synchronous pressure-flow cystourethrography became established as a result of these advances[18] and these studies provide both visual and pressure recordings of the changes in the bladder and the urethra during voiding. On filling the bladder, the presence of any leakage into the urethra may be noted and provocative tests, such as standing, coughing or straining will show the competence of the mechanism at the bladder neck. When the detrusor contracts on voiding, the behaviour of the bladder neck can be noted, so that any imbalance or dyssynergia between detrusor contraction and proximal urethral relaxation can be assessed and the site of any obstruction accurately localised.

If the patient is asked to stop in mid-stream whilst voiding, the closing mechanism of the urethra may be observed. In a person with normal function this closure of the urethra can be accomplished in about 0.25 sec. Interruption of the urinary stream is established by contraction of the peri-urethral striated muscle of the pelvic floor, inhibition of detrusor contraction and the urethral closure follows with a milk-back effect of radio-opaque dye into the bladder on bladder neck closure.

Electromyographic studies of the pelvic floor have added yet further sophistication to the investigations of lower urinary tract function.

Porter[19] showed that the pelvic floor muscles were unique in showing continuous activity even when at rest (see Chapter 4, p. 79). This EMG activity is increased when intra-abdominal pressure is raised, but is absent during voiding. Thomas *et al.*[20] demonstrated the value of these studies in patients with neurological lesions, particularly those who have an abnormality of the balance between detrusor and sphincter mechanisms, or so-termed detrusor sphincteric dyssynergia.

The Definitions of Urinary Incontinence

The foregoing account has outlined some of the mechanisms associated with the normal storage and voiding of urine in the micturition cycle. Urinary incontinence denotes a failure of these, so that involuntary leakage of urine occurs in inappropriate places or at inappropriate times. The Standardisation Committee of the International Continence Society (ICS) has defined incontinence as a condition in which the involuntary loss of urine is a social or hygienic problem and is objectively demonstrable. Loss of urine through channels other than the urethra is termed extra-urethral incontinence and this includes the congenital abnormalities, such as ectopia vesicae and the loss of urine through vesical, ureteric or urethral fistulae. One of the major problems with all definitions of incontinence is the variable threshold at which the individual considers it to be a problem. The occasional loss of urine to one person may be an inconvenience, whereas to another it is a disaster.

A classification of the types of incontinence, based on their clinical presentation, does provide a framework which assists identification of the possible cause. It enables the clinician at least to place the problem in a provisional group, so that an appropriate and selective course of clinical evaluation may follow.

Stress Incontinence

Stress incontinence may be considered a symptom, a sign or a condition. The symptom is associated with the involuntary loss of urine that occurs on coughing, laughing, sneezing or any physical exertion.

The sign of stress incontinence is the observation of urinary loss from the urethra, when the patient is asked to raise intra-abdominal pressure by coughing or straining. It is not always possible to demonstrate this with the patient in the dorsal position, but it is worth asking the patient to stand up and to cough again, so long as the carpet is protected.

The condition of genuine stress incontinence, as defined by the ICS is the involuntary loss of urine that occurs when intravesical pressure exceeds the maximum urethral pressure, in the absence of a detrusor contraction. This is a definition based on urodynamic parameters and it is important because some patients, on coughing or straining, will stimulate a detrusor contraction that will present as 'stress incontinence'. The distinction between the patient with a stable detrusor with genuine stress incontinence and the patient with an unstable detrusor is an important factor in the pre-operative assessment of this group. Stress incontinence is associated with a defect in the urethral sphincter mechanism, when the detrusor activity is normal (see Chapter 3, p. 55).

Urge Incontinence

Urge incontinence is the involuntary loss of urine associated with a strong desire to void. It has been subdivided into motor urge incontinence, when it is related to unstable detrusor contractions on cystometry, and sensory urge incontinence, when the hypersensitivity of the bladder and urethral sensory receptors prevents normal filling of the bladder. In clinical practice, motor urge incontinence is more commonly a problem and, although sensory urge may be associated with pathological changes in the lower urinary tract, such as infection or stones, it is less commonly a cause for incontinence.

Overflow Incontinence

Retention with overflow is a well-recognised clinical condition. The incontinence occurs when the intravesical pressure exceeds the maximum urethral pressure. Long-standing obstruction causes distension of the bladder, which reaches the limit of its compliance. Effective detrusor contraction is prevented and leakage of urine arises. The raised intravesical pressure may cause obstruction to the upper urinary tract and impairment of renal function. The common cause for the problem is prostatic obstruction, due to hyperplasia or carcinoma. It must always be carefully distinguished from those cases in which a detrusor failure is related to a neurological abnormality. Lesions of the cauda equina, a diabetic neuropathy or rarely, tabes dorsalis, may present in this way. Faecal impaction is another common cause (see Chapter 4).

Enuresis

The strict definition of enuresis is incontinence of urine, but it is usually used to describe bed-wetting. Nocturnal enuresis is a more accurate term for this condition, in order to distinguish the problem from the less common diurnal enuresis of some schoolchildren. Primary nocturnal enuresis is used to differentiate those children with lifelong bed-wetting from secondary or late-onset enuresis, which arises after a period of complete control.

Although the majority of enuretic children are dry by the age of puberty, a few continue into early adult life and a high proportion of these have been shown to have unstable bladders on urodynamic investigation. Whiteside and Arnold[21] reviewed 50 patients referred to their unit for investigation and distinguished 13 with nocturnal enuresis alone and 37 with diurnal-nocturnal enuresis. Two out of the 13 patients with the problem of bed-wetting had unstable bladders, whilst 36 out of the 37 with the diurnal-nocturnal enuresis had unstable bladders. In a study of 54 adult enuretics, Torrens and Collins[22] showed bladder instability in 70 per cent of the patients and obstruction of micturition in only six per cent.

Continuous Incontinence

Continuous dribbling incontinence may be subdivided into those cases where the patient is conscious of the problem and those where it is an unconscious loss. Conscious and continuous dribbling incontinence is in fact a rare condition and it is most often related to a reduced urethral resistance caused by sphincter damage or degenerative changes. A small bladder capacity is a rare cause for dribbling incontinence.

Unconscious continuous incontinence is usually related to a neurological abnormality.

Post-micturition Dribbling

It is not uncommon for young and older men to seek advice regarding this problem of the post-micturition dribble of urine. The complaint is usually described as a slight loss that occurs when they walk away from the toilet, but it stains the underwear and if they are wearing tight trousers may be observed on these. In the young man, it is usually related to a failure of the bulbo spongiosum muscle to evacuate the bulb of the urethra, but the cause for this is not apparent. It may follow a urethritis or urethral instrumentation and in most cases it responds rapidly to the advice to compress the urethral bulb manually at the end of micturition. In the older man, the condition can follow prostatectomy or it may be related to early outflow obstruction. Whiteside has described the trapping of urine that can arise in some cases between the proximal and urethral sphincter mechanisms at the termination of voiding. As the distal mechanism relaxes, urine escapes. In women, it is not a common problem, but occasionally urine pools in the vagina during micturition and then escapes after completion of the act.

Notes

1. Donker, P.J., Dröes, J. Tu P.M. and van Ulden, B.M. (1976), 'Anatomy of the Musculature and Innervation of the Bladder and the Urethra' in Innes Williams, D. and Chisholm, G.D. (eds.), *Scientific Foundation of Urology, vol. II* (Heinemann, London), 32-8.

2. Gosling, J.A. (1979), 'The Structure of the Bladder and Urethra in Relation to Function', *Urol. Clin. North America, 6*, 31-8.

3. Hutch, J.A. (1965), 'A New Theory of the Anatomy of the Internal Sphincter and the Phsyiology of Micturition', *Inv. Urol., 3*, 36-58.

4. Jeffcoate, T.N.A. and Roberts, H. (1952), 'Stress Incontinence of Urine, 2', *J. Obstet. Gynaec. Brit. Emp., 59*, 685-720.

5. Smith, P. (1972), 'Age Changes in the Female Urethra', *Brit. J. Urol., 44*, 667-76.

6. Turner Warwick, R. (1979), 'Observations on the Function and Dysfunction of the Sphincter and Detrusor Mechanisms', *Urol. Clin. North America, 6*, 13-30.

7. Nathan, P.W. (1976), 'The Central Nervous Connections of the Bladder' in Innes Williams, D. and Chisholm, G.D. (eds.), *Scientific Foundations of Urology, vol. II* (Heinemann, London), 51-8.

8. Hess, W.R. (1957), in Hughes, J.P. (ed.), *The Functional Organization of the Diencephalon* (Grune and Stratton, New York and London).

9. Brown, M. and Wickham, J.E.A. (1969), 'The Urethral Pressure Profile', *Brit. J. Urol., 41*, 211-17.

10. Abrams, P.H. (1979), 'Perfusion Urethral Profilometry', *Urol. Clin. North America, 6*, 103-9.

11. Enhorning, G. (1961), 'Simultaneous Recording of Intravesical and Intraurethral Pressure', *Acta Chir. Scand. Suppl., 276*, 1-68.

12. Bates, C.P. (1971), 'Continence and Incontinence: A Clinical Study of the Dynamics of Voiding and of the Sphincter Mechanism', *Ann. Roy. Coll. Surg. Eng., 49*, 18-35.

13. Von Garrelts, B. (1956), 'Analysis of Micturition. A New Method of Recording the Voiding of the Bladder', *Acta. Chir. Scand., 112*, 326-40.

14. Abrams, P.H. and Torrens, M.J. (1979), 'Urine Flow Studies', *Urol. Clin. North America, 6*, 71-9.

15. Muellner, S.R. (1949), 'Physiologic Components of Urinary Bladder: Their Clinical Significance', *New Engl. J. Med., 241*, 769-72.

16. Hinman, F.J., Miller, G.M., Nickel, E. and Miller, E.R. (1954), 'Vesical Physiology Demonstrated by Cine-radiography and Serial Roentgenography: Preliminary Report', *Radiology, 62*, 713-19.

17. Tanagho, E.A., Meyers, F.H. and Smith, D.R. (1969), 'Urethral Resistance: Its Components and Implications i. Smooth Muscle Component ii. Striated Muscle Component', *Inv. Urol., 7*, 136-49 (September) and 195-205 (November).

18. Bates, C.P., Whiteside, C.G. and Turner Warwick, R. (1970), 'Synchronous Cine/Pressure/Flow/Cysto-urethrography with Special Reference to Stress and Urge Incontinence', *Brit. J. Urol., 42*, 714-23.

19. Porter, N.H. (1962), 'A Physiological Study of the Pelvic Floor in Rectal Prolapse', *Ann. Roy. Coll. Surg. Eng., 31*, 379-404.

20. Thomas, D.G., Smallwood, R. and Graham, D. (1975), 'Urodynamic

Observations Following Spinal Trauma', *Brit. J. Urol., 47*, 161-75.

21.   Whiteside, C.G. and Arnold, E.P. (1975), 'Persistent Primary Enuresis. A Urodynamic Assessment', *Brit. Med. J., 1*, 364-7.

22.   Torrens, M.J. and Collins, C.D. (1975), 'The Urodynamic Assessment of Adult Enuresis', *Brit. J. Urol., 47*, 433-40.

2 UROLOGICAL ASPECTS OF INCONTINENCE

Roger C.L. Feneley

Patients seek medical advice regarding urinary incontinence for three main reasons. First, they fear the prospect of losing bladder control, secondly they may have experienced an isolated incidence of incontinence and thirdly, they may have established incontinence which they have attempted to hide or stoically accept until their morale has finally succumbed.

The spectrum of incontinence is wide and as the development of a clinical service improves, so more patients are attracted to seek advice and treatment. In a survey of 4,211 young nulliparous nursing students, Wolin[1] reported that 50.7 per cent had some degree of stress incontinence and 16 per cent on a daily basis, but none of these had ever sought medical attention, either because they felt ashamed of admitting it or they felt this was not abnormal. This study confirmed the earlier survey of Nemir and Middleton[2] which reported a 52 per cent incidence of stress incontinence amongst 1,300 college girls, with 5 per cent experiencing the problem on a regular basis. The prevalance of incontinence in the community is a relevant factor, but its accurate estimation is difficult, not only because of the practical aspects of collecting meaningful data, but also due to the variable threshold of its recognition. In a survey of recognised incontinence in a population of 37,000 in the Bristol area, reports received from general practitioners, community nurses, social and welfare services revealed a prevalence of one per cent. To estimate the unrecognised prevalence, a postal survey was undertaken in one group practice of 7,500 patients near Bristol and compared with an identical survey undertaken in Harrow. Thomas[3] (see Chapter 14) reported these findings and showed that eight per cent of women aged 15-64 years experienced incontinence twice or more per month. Many of these patients, however, accept this inconvenience and do not consider medical advice necessary.

Urinary incontinence amongst geriatric patients raises both economic and management problems. Exton-Smith[4] showed that 25 per cent of nursing time on a geriatric ward was spent dealing with incontinent patients and the high proportion of patients with cerebrovascular disease and brain loss of one type or another, necessitates adequate palliative measures with suitable appliances, rather than operative treatment (see Chapter 6A). The development of a urodynamic unit in the Urology Department in Bristol has emphasised the problems of urinary incontinence. Some 2,290 patients were investigated between 1975 and 1979 and of these 1,596 (70 per cent) had some degree of incontinence. There were 758 men and 54 per cent had some incontinence. The majority of these had either urge incontinence (33 per cent), enuresis (25 per cent) or a post-micturition dribble (27 per cent). Out of a total of 1,532 women 70 per cent had urinary incontinence and the most common types were stress incontinence (25 per cent), stress and urge incontinence (33 per cent), urge incontinence (20 per cent) and enuresis (10 per cent). Continuous incontinence, either conscious or unconscious, was present in 10 per cent of the men and 8 per cent of the women (see Table 2.1). The grade of incontinence showed differences between the male and female groups. Although 42 per cent of the men noticed some soiling of their clothes, only 5 per cent wore any protective padding. This compared with 45 per cent of the women who wet their clothes and 36 per cent who used some form of protection.[5]

Table 2.1: Types of Incontinence

	Male (%)	Female (%)
Stress	2	25
Stress/Urge	1	33
Urge	33	20
Enuresis	25	10
Post-Micturition dribble	27	1
Continuous	10	8
Uncategorised	2	3

The Initial Clinical Assessment

The assessment of the patient with urinary incontinence demands a methodical approach, starting with a careful history to identify the type, duration, severity and any relevant precipitating factors. Urodynamic investigations, particularly those employing synchronous video-pressure flow cystourethrography, have re-emphasised the value of the history by correlating the patient's symptoms with the appearance and the behaviour in mechanical terms of the bladder and urethra during filling and voiding. It has made possible the analysis of the symptoms according to the state of detrusor activity or urethral sphincter function.

Incontinence that occurs only on coughing, laughing, sneezing or walking and is unassociated with any other urinary symptoms is termed 'stress incontinence' and under such circumstances, 90 per cent of the patients will have a stable bladder which fills at a low pressure below 15 cm of water and shows no evidence of detrusor contraction. The actual urine loss in these cases tends to be small on each occasion.

Frequency, urgency with urge incontinence amounting to episodes of flooding at times, implies detrusor instability. Whiteside[6] showed that 80 per cent of women with urge incontinence had unstable bladders and he defined frequency as the act of micturition which was necessary at least every two hours during the day and the arousal from sleep by the desire to void regularly once or twice every night. However, the symptoms of stress and urge incontinence may be combined and the differentiation of these two groups requires specialised investigation.

Overflow incontinence is typified by the middle-aged or elderly man with chronic retention, who starts wetting the bed at night or finds that he is wet without any sensation of the need to void. This problem is related to bladder outflow obstruction and in some cases may be associated with the symptoms of early renal failure, such as an increasing thirst, loss of appetite and taste or breathlessness and anginal pain from the associated anaemia. Overflow incontinence, related to neurological lesions, can usually be suspected from the history. Continuous dribbling incontinence can imply a serious pathological or structural abnormality. The onset may be related to major trauma or pelvic surgery, such as hysterectomy or abdomino-perineal resection, when pelvic nerve damage may be implicated.[7] Extra-urethral incontinence from fistulae also falls into this category. The young girl with an ectopic ureter entering the vagina is a rare problem, but should be suspected if the incontinence is continuous.

The grade of incontinence can be judged by the remedial action which has become necessary. In men staining of the underwear or trousers is often the major cause for concern, particularly from their wives, but women may need to change underclothes or wear pads. The number of changes per day or week is a helpful guide to this assessment.

A detailed history may not be possible in patients with impairment of cerebral function. A simple mental acuity test can often reveal a degree of dementia that would not otherwise have been suspected, particularly if the patient is brought to the clinic by a caring relative. Gross exaggeration of the symptoms is not uncommon amongst patients with serious emotional disturbances.

Many patients receive drugs for conditions, such as peptic ulceration, hypertension or bronchospasm, which can have a secondary effect on lower urinary tract function. A careful note should be taken of these, particularly if they have an anticholinergic or sympathomimetic effect. Diuretics are also frequently prescribed and many patients do not appreciate their specific action.

The Physical Examination

Observation of the patient's mobility and dexterity can raise suspicion of an otherwise unsuspected neurological disorder and it also provides a useful indication of the patient's suitability for operative treatment that may later be under consideration. His ability to climb on to the examination couch and a record of the pulse and blood pressure will normally reveal any serious cardiorespiratory problem.

Abdominal examination may expose the distended bladder of chronic retention, but obesity and an atonic detrusor muscle may make it difficult to recognise in some cases. In addition uterine or ovarian swellings need careful differentiation.

Inspection of the perineum, particularly the skin around the scrotum or vulva, not forgetting the state of the underclothes, can indicate the severity of the incontinence. Rectal examination not only provides information regarding the presence of pathology in the anal canal, lower rectum and pelvis, but it gives the opportunity to assess peri-anal and anal sensation, anal tone and the presence of any faecal impaction. In the male the size of the prostate gland is noted, but its consistency, particularly regarding any irregularity or loss of the median sulcus suggesting carcinoma, is far more important. An enlarged prostate is not necessarily associated with outflow obstruction.

The vaginal examination should be undertaken in any position with which the clinician is familiar and which will allow thorough inspection of the vulva. The position of the external urethral meatus and its appearance, as well as that of the labia, should be noted and evidence of atrophic vaginitis or discharge recorded. The appearance of urethral mucosal prolapse, confined to the posterior border of the urethra, can readily be confused with that of a urethral caruncle, but the latter is exquisitely tender to touch. On asking the patient to cough, the presence of anterior vaginal wall or uterine prolapse should be observed. In patients with stress incontinence, a spurt of urine may be seen, particularly if the coughing is repeated. Palpation of the vagina with the finger may indicate urethral tenderness in patients with urethritis and, on asking the patient to draw up or tighten the vagina, the strength of the pubo-vaginal contraction gives some impression of the voluntary control over the pelvic floor muscles. It can be helpful if one explains how these muscles function at this stage of the examination. Just as one notes the state of the anal tone on rectal examination, so vaginal tone should be examined, as many women have no idea that voluntary control of these muscles ever exists. The pelvic examination is completed with a bimanual palpation and a speculum to inspect the cervix and fornices.

A full neurological examination should be performed if there is any sensory loss in the perineal area which is supplied by the sacral nerves, or a defect in anal tone. The knee jerk (L4), ankle jerk (S1) and plantar reflexes can readily be tested and inspection of the spine excludes the pad of hair or dimple that may be associated with spinal dysraphism.

Examination of the Urine

Urinalysis is a routine part of any clinical examination. The finding of proteinuria or glycosuria may account for disturbances of micturition and diabetes mellitus can be associated with a peripheral neuropathy that affects detrusor and urethral function. Any positive findings clearly require full and appropriate investigation.

The collection of a mid-stream specimen of urine, and its delivery to and plating-out in the pathology laboratory, require careful consideration and the final report requires a critical analysis. The urine sample is likely to be contaminated before ever reaching the sterile container, if the male patient has a tight phimosis or, in the case of the female, if she is grossly obese or if she has a vaginal discharge. It can be particularly difficult for the elderly patient, of either sex, especially if bedbound, to provide a clean-catch specimen, and under such circumstances, two or three specimens should be sent for examination. When the specimen has been collected, it should either be plated-out in the laboratory within the hour or placed immediately in a refrigerator at 4°C until a quick delivery to the laboratory is undertaken. Most urinary pathogens multiply rapidly at room temperature and undue delay in this delivery service can give misleading results.

The report of the microscopy and culture result should be accepted with caution. The vast majority of patients with symptomatic infection have significant pyuria, but pyuria is a non-specific finding and patients *with and without pyuria may or may not have infection.* It is usually accepted that a clean-catch specimen of urine showing more than 100,000 (10^5) organisms/ml is consistent with a significant urinary tract infection, but in an *asymptomatic* female, there is an 80 per cent probability only that this presents a true bacteriuria.[8] If two separate specimens demonstrate at least 10^5 of the same bacteria/ml, the probability increases to 95 per cent. Thus, it is necessary in some cases to repeat the MSU investigation. *Proteus* organisms do not produce a rapid growth and the demonstration of these organisms in counts of less than 10^5 bacteria/ml should always raise the possibility of calculus disease in the urinary tract. Pyuria alone should raise suspicion of possible urinary tract tuberculosis, calculi or a urethral stricture.

When urine specimens cannot be delivered rapidly to the laboratory, the use of the dip-inoculum slide is to be recommended. The slide is dipped in the urinary stream during voiding and this may then be sent by post to the laboratory for analysis.

The misuse of broad-spectrum antibiotic therapy for doubtful urinary tract infection, not only misleads the patient but exposes him or her to the hazard of sensitivity reactions and, in the case of women, the possibility of a monilial vaginitis.

The Frequency/Volume Chart

A simple guide to micturition disorders may be obtained by the use of a frequency/volume chart that is recorded by the patient (see Figure 2.1).

Figure 2.1: Example of a Simple Frequency/Volume Chart

Day	Time/volume (ml)					
	Daytime				Nightime	
1	7am/200	1pm/−*	6pm/400	11pm/300	3am/200	6am/w**
2						
3						

*   At work, could not measure volume.
** Wet at 6am.

Using any appropriate measure, such as that employed in the kitchen, the patient is asked to note the time and the volume passed on voiding for 24-hour periods whenever this is convenient. It provides details of the actual frequency experienced by the patient, exposing any exaggeration in their original history, and also gives a measure of their maximum functional bladder capacity. The first specimen of urine passed in the morning often gives this measurement of overnight capacity. It is not unusual for a volume of 350-400 ml to be passed in the morning, only to be followed by a record showing volumes of 50-150 ml during the day. Such a chart usually signifies a psychological problem. This is in marked contrast to the patient who never passes more than 200 ml at a time and who requires to void two or three times at night.

The chart also differentiates those patients who have an alteration in circadian rhythm. Amongst some elderly patients more urine is passed during the night than during the day and this readily accounts for the nocturia which they experience.

Episodes of incontinence are also recorded on the chart. In practice, these records have been maintained extremely accurately by patients and they can give rise to considerable motivation when they realise that their functional bladder capacity is within the normal range.

Primary Clinical Management

Urinary incontinence is rarely an isolated problem, but is more often just one aspect of a systemic disorder. Obesity, chronic cough, excessive drinking with polyuria may be associated problems (see Chapter 5, p. 101). The initial assessment should provide a provisional diagnosis on which the general practitioner can base his further policy, but whereas accurate diagnosis is the clinician's major prerogative, *advice and early treatment are the patient's greatest concern.*

A history of urinary incontinence, associated with haematuria, the demonstration of abnormal physical signs or the findings of a chronic urinary tract infection will clearly necessitate referral for specialist advice and investigation. In the absence of any demonstrable structural or pathological abnormality, a psychosomatic problem may be unveiled, for which immediate referral to hospital may *not* be in the patient's best interest. Particular care should be taken with the patient who has been recently bereaved. Nor does a hospital referral answer the problem of the soiled linen and the additional laundering costs that create so much distress to the patient or relatives. The management presents a challenge and a broad knowledge of the measures and supportive aids outlined later in this book is invaluable. In one family of five children, four of whom were enuretic, the divorced mother was persuaded not to leave home by the local authority, who provided her with a washing machine.

Urge incontinence accounts for about 30 per cent of patients referred to gynaecological clinics[9] and is a common problem amongst elderly patients. The irritable bladder syndrome, presenting with frequency, urgency and urge incontinence, may be cured by irradication of a urinary tract infection or the symptoms may respond to drug therapy. Failure to respond, however, should not warrant despair, but merely underlines the need for further investigation.

Minor degrees of stress incontinence have already been mentioned as a common problem in women and many patients accept the occasional inconvenience as a normal hazard. Instruction in pelvic floor control can be of assistance to some patients in this group, who have no significant cystocoele or uterine prolapse. The continuous unremitting incontinence of the debilitated or geriatric patient can be treated by means of a suitable appliance or catheter, but their management requires a knowledgeable clinician and nurse to supervise them adequately.

Between these extremes, there are patients who will require referral to a hospital clinic for specialist advice, but this can prolong the patient's distress yet further. A trial of drug treatment or pelvic floor exercises and advice on protective garments should not be dismissed as a waste of time.

Drug Treatment

A wide range of drugs are now available, which can influence detrusor and urethral smooth muscle activity. Unfortunately, the results of treatment are variable and their side-effects can be unpleasant so that the patient cannot tolerate a full course. In such cases, suitable alternative drugs should be considered.

The rationale of drug therapy is based on the innervation of the lower tract by parasympathetic cholinergic fibres and the sympathetic supply with a concentration of alpha-adrenergic receptors around the proximal urethra and the presence of beta-adrenergic receptors in the fundus of the bladder.

Drugs with a cholinergic effect stimulate detrusor contraction, whilst those with an anticholinergic action reduce its contractility. Alpha-adrenergic preparations stimulate contraction of the proximal urethra, whilst alpha-blocking drugs relax this region. Beta-adrenergic drugs relax the detrusor and beta-blockers may increase detrusor contractility.

Cholinergic Drugs

Cholinergic drugs are most frequently used post-operatively in patients with an underactive detrusor, to re-establish spontaneous voiding after surgery, or in selected patients with neurogenic bladder problems. They have a limited place in routine practice and should be avoided in patients with bladder outflow obstruction. Carbachol may be administered subcutaneously 0.25-0.5 mg, orally 1-4 mg prn, and bethanechol (Myotonine) in dosage of 2-5 mg subcutaneously or 5-30 mg orally. The anticholinesterase preparation distigmine (Ubretid) has a similar action and can be given i.m. 0.5 mg or orally 5 mg daily, but it is extremely expensive. These cholinergic drugs can cause severe side reactions, with profuse sweating, lacrimation or gastro-intestinal colic and should be used with caution.

Anticholinergic drugs

These drugs can be of value in patients with irritable or unstable bladders. They act at the post-ganglionic nerve endings, with an atropine-like action or at the site of ganglionic transmission. Propantheline (Probanthine) 15-30 mg t.d.s. can increase the bladder capacity, if the detrusor is compliant, but effective dosage may cause a dry mouth and temporary loss of visual accommodation. Emepronium bromide (Cetiprin) in adequate dosage of 200 mg q.d.s. is useful, but can cause a dry mouth and tachycardia.

Imipramine (Tofranil) 25-50 mg t.d.s. has anticholinergic properties, but in addition it blocks the re-uptake of noradrenaline, thus sensitising the alpha-adrenergic receptors at the bladder neck, promoting its closure.

Probanthine, Cetiprin and imipramine should be given a trial in patients with urge incontinence, due to detrusor overactivity. Urispas, 200 mg q.d.s. has also been recommended as an antispasmodic musculotrophic preparation and Stanton[10] showed a beneficial effect in patients with frequency, stress and urge incontinence.

Alpha-adrenergic Agonist

Ephedrine, 15-30 mg t.d.s. is used in the relief of bronchospasm, but it can promote retention of urine by stimulating proximal urethral closure.

Alpha-adrenergic Antagonist

Phenoxybenzamine is of value in patients with poor voiding ability, due to neurogenic disorders of bladder function. Scott and Morrow[11] used phenoxybenzamine in doses of 10-60 mg daily in patients with spinal cord injuries with good effect and it also has a place in the management of children with myelomeningocoele.

Beta-adrenergic Agonists

Orciprenaline (Alupent) 20 mg q.d.s. or salbutamol (Ventolin) 2-4 mg t.d.s. may be used in patients with bladder instability. Orciprenaline in combination with emepronium has also been recommended in this group.

Pelvic Floor Exercises

Kegel[12] advocated physiologic therapy in women with stress incontinence and considered that some of the most gratifying results were obtained in debilitated elderly women. He used a perineometer (see Appendix to Chapter 10) to measure the patient's ability to squeeze an air-filled balloon placed in the vagina, in order to register the strength of the pelvic muscles. In a series of 500 cases of stress incontinence, 75 per cent of the women who initially had partial control of these muscles experienced complete relief of symptoms after a seven to eight week course of pelvic floor exercises. In those with cystocoele or uterine prolapse requiring surgery, Kegel recommended these exercises during the pre-operative and post-operative management. Hoffman and Sokol[13] and Jones[14] have also advised this form of treatment in patients with stress incontinence.

In our unit, Shepherd and Montgomery showed significant improvement in 21 out of 22 patients with stress incontinence receiving intensive re-education of the pelvic floor, so that the patients no longer considered they had a problem (see Chapter 10). Frequency of micturition and nocturia were also diminished and the beneficial response could be monitored by use of the perineometer.

Moore and Schofield[15] used pelvic floor faradism under general anaesthesia for the treatment of stress incontinence in women. They reported 10 out of 18 patients with stress incontinence were either considerably or completely relieved of their symptoms by this treatment. Although four patients relapsed during the initial six months following treatment, two of them responded to further faradism and the other two did not consider their symptoms warranted treatment. Collins[16] and Shepherd[17] in our unit have used this treatment at the time of cystoscopy under general anaesthesia in a total of 107 patients and reported a cure rate of 23 per cent and 30 per cent respectively, with a follow-up period of one year. A long-term follow-up is clearly indicated to fully evaluate these results.

Urological Aspects of Management

There is considerable overlap of interest in the problems of incontinent patients between the urologist and the gynaecologist and this has been emphasised by the introduction of urodynamic investigations. The ageing process tends to increase the sphincteric resistance of the outflow tract in men, whereas in women sphincteric resistance tends to decrease and may be associated with cystocoele or a uterine prolapse (see Chapter 3, p. 58). In both men and women, urinary symptoms can be associated with detrusor instability and in men this may arise as a secondary feature of outflow obstruction. It is important to differentiate between those patients with or without evidence of obstruction, because patients with detrusor instability without demonstrable obstruction tend not to benefit from operative treatment to the outflow tract. Urodynamic investigations in the male have provided objective evidence of the presence of obstruction. In a series of 318 patients between the ages of 45 and 84, symptoms suggestive of bladder outflow obstruction were investigated by urodynamic studies. In 33 per cent of the patients, no evidence of obstruction was demonstrable and surgery was thus avoided.[18]

The urological assessment of urinary tract disorders includes selective investigations by means of biochemical, radiological, urodynamic and endoscopic means.

Biochemical Investigation

Serum creatinine estimation (normal range 90-120 mcmol/1) is a more sensitive estimation of renal function than that of the blood urea (normal range 3.0-7.0 mcmol/1). Long-standing renal impairment is usually associated with anaemia.

Radiological Investigation

The simplest radiological investigation is the straight X-ray of the urinary tract. This identifies any urinary calculi and may also give an estimate of the size of the soft tissue shadow of the bladder. Particularly in patients who have had previous urological surgery or who have had an indwelling catheter for a period of time following severe skeletal injuries, for example, it is important to exclude the possible development of a bladder calculus, which may account for persistent urinary symptoms and incontinence (see Figure 2.2).

Figure 2.2: A Straight Radiograph of the Urinary Tract Showing a Calculus in an Elderly Patient with Urge Incontinence

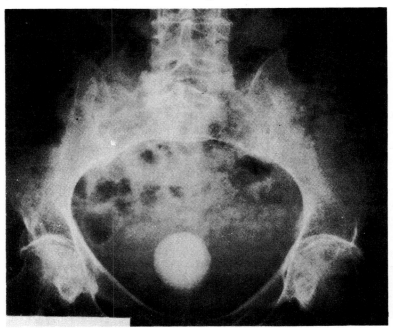

The excretion urogram or intravenous pyelogram (IVP) is the routine investigation to demonstrate the anatomy of the upper urinary tract. It also provides evidence of the size, shape and thickness of the bladder and can give an estimate of the residual urine following voiding. This assessment of the residual urine, however, can be very misleading and interpretation in terms of obstruction should be cautious.

Micturating Cystourethrography (MCUG)

Bladder function has been studied by using contrast medium to fill the bladder by a catheter, but the value of this investigation depends on the particular experience and interest of the radiologist. The MCUG is used to demonstrate vesico-ureteric reflux, but its place in the study of bladder function has been surpassed by the introduction of synchronous video pressure-flow cystourethrography.

Urodynamic Investigations

The information provided by urodynamic investigations has already been outlined in the previous chapter. The basic investigations consist of:

(1) urine flow studies;
(2) filling and voiding cystometrography;
(3) the urethral pressure profile in selective problems; and
(4) synchronous pressure-flow cystourethrography with video-recording.

Evaluation of urodynamic investigations gives assessment of bladder sensation, together with detrusor and sphincter functions. The detrusor activity may be classified as normal, hyperactive or hypoactive and sphincter resistance may be normal, increased or decreased. The synchronous video pressure-flow cystourethrography provides the most sophisticated method of analysing bladder and urethral function and it displays the appearance of the bladder and urethra during filling and voiding. The competence of the bladder neck mechanisms can be evaluated by asking the patient to cough, strain or stand when the bladder is filled and, during voiding, abnormalities of the outflow tract may be visualised. However, the equipment is expensive and for the most practical purposes routine pressure-flow studies and the urethral pressure profile are very satisfactory (see Figures 2.3, 2.4 and 2.5, and Chapter 3).

Endoscopic Examination

Direct visualisation of the bladder and urethra identifies such problems as urethral strictures, bladder neoplasm and calculi. By performing the examination under general anaesthesia, a measure of the bladder capacity can be recorded and the problems of the contracted bladder can be recognised. The appearance of bladder trabeculation is associated with a hyperactive detrusor, but this is not synonymous with obstruction.

Endoscopic examination as an investigation is ideally reserved as the final urological assessment. If the functional studies have shown evidence of obstruction, the endoscopic examination excludes unsuspected pathology in the bladder and can make a final assessment of the outflow tract, so that operative treatment can proceed without further delay, either by transurethral or retropubic methods.

In patients with evidence of a small functional bladder capacity, endoscopy does evaluate the true anatomical capacity and, in selected patients, bladder distension using hydrostatic or balloon distension by the Helmstein method[19] may be used.

Figure 2.3: A Recording of the Urine Flow Before Prostatectomy

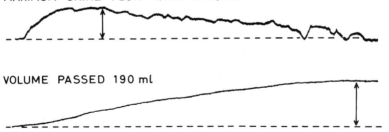

MAXIMUM URINE FLOW RATE 6ml/sec

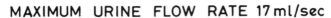

VOLUME PASSED 190 ml

Figure 2.4: Urine Flow After Prostatectomy

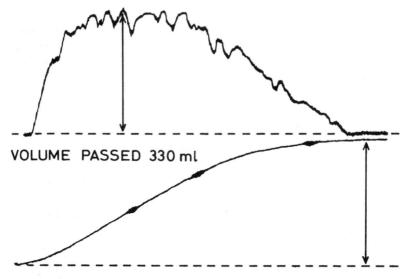

MAXIMUM URINE FLOW RATE 17 ml/sec

VOLUME PASSED 330 ml

Figure 2.5: The Urethral Pressure Profile Before and After Prostatectomy

PREOPERATIVE   POSTOPERATIVE

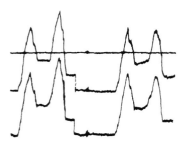 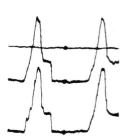

Maximum Perineal Stimulation (MPS)

This has been used in patients with both urge and stress incontinence. The treatment is at present under trial, but it is based on the suggestion that vaginal or rectal electrode stimulation of the pelvic floor can produce relaxation of the detrusor muscle.[20] The value of MPS in patients with stress incontinence has already been mentioned.

Urological Management of Incontinence

Sensory Urge Incontinence

In a small proportion of these patients, investigation does reveal pathological abnormalities, such as an acute or chronic urinary tract infection, urinary calculi, bladder tumours or a small contracted bladder. The contracted bladder may be related to interstitial cystitis, a systolic bladder associated with tuberculous infection, or a post-radiation fibrosis. Bladder distension, using the Helmstein balloon method, as already mentioned, has an application in the treatment of interstitial cystitis and enterocystoplasty, employing a patch of bowel from ileum or colon to enlarge the bladder capacity, has application in selected patients with detrusor fibrosis. Urinary diversion, using an ileal or colon conduit, may be necessary in severe cases.

Motor Urge Incontinence

This is related to the failure of cortical inhibition of detrusor contraction and cystometrography demonstrates an unstable detrusor. It may arise secondary to bladder outflow obstruction and in these cases relief of the obstruction will alleviate the problem. However, a wide range of problems remains, such as the enuretic group of patients particularly those with diurnal and nocturnal symptoms, and a high proportion of elderly incontinent patients. A variety of measures has been advocated for the treatment of this group, measures such as transection of the bladder,[21] selective sacral neurectomy[22] and Helmstein distension,[19] but the results of treatment are variable. A psychosomatic approach to the problem has been advocated[9] and a more conservative approach to this group has arisen with the use of bio-feedback techniques.[23] (see Chapter 3, p. 72).

Overflow Incontinence

In patients with bladder outflow obstruction, conventional measures, such as transurethral resection of the bladder neck and prostrate gland or retropubic prostatectomy, are undertaken. A small proportion of these patients have neurogenic bladders and particular caution needs to be exercised with these.

The Neurogenic Bladder

The management of patients with neurological disorders affecting the bladder is an extremely complex and specialised field. It includes a very wide range of disorders, which affect the brain or spinal cord. Multiple sclerosis may present with urinary symptoms and Desmond and Shuttleworth[24] advocated early consideration of urinary diversion in this group.

Patients with spinal cord lesions have received particular attention with the development of spinal injury units. The life expectancy in these patients is directly related to the maintenance of renal function, which can be readily impaired by the development of an obstructive uropathy as a result of the dyssynergia or imbalance between the detrusor and the sphincter. Upper tract dilatation with vesico-ureteric reflux and pyelonephritis can be a major threat to their prognosis. Similar problems arise amongst children with myelomeningocoele. The vital principles of management include first the establishment of satisfactory bladder emptying, with the avoidance of an indwelling catheter, secondly, the maintenance of normal upper urinary tracts and thirdly, the maintenance of a sterile urine.[25] The management of the associated urinary incontinence is particularly important, owing to the risk of severe pressure sores in this group. Male patients may be managed by means of appliances such as the condom sheath, but there is no satisfactory appliance for female patients. Urinary diversion may need to be considered. Intermittent self-catheterisation[26, 27] also has a place in the management of selected cases.

Post-prostatectomy Incontinence

Temporary loss of urine control following prostatic surgery is not uncommon. After relief of obstruction at the bladder neck and prostatic urethra, a weak distal sphincter may be the sole mechanism for the maintenance of continence. This usually recovers within the first week after surgery and the patient is encouraged to practise stopping and starting micturition during voiding, in order to exercise the voluntary pelvic muscles. Continued incontinence may be related to residual obstruction, an unstable bladder or a damaged sphincter and careful evaluation of these is necessary.

When the distal sphincter mechanism is damaged, slow improvement may arise during the first few months after surgery. However, continued incontinence requires treatment and various implanted devices are now available. Kaufman[28] introduced a method of urethral compression using a silicone envelope, which is implanted over the bulbar urethra and attached to the ischio-pubic rami with straps. He reported a 62 per cent cure-rate with this method. Scott *et al.*[29] and Rosen[30] have both introduced inflatable occluding devices, which can be implanted around the urethra. The most encouraging results have been obtained in patients with post-prostatectomy incontinence and the development of implantable artificial sphincters could provide a valuable contribution.

Caldwell[31] first used an electrical implant for treating urinary incontinence in 1963 and since then this method has been used in a number of specialist centres. Mechanical problems with the electrodes can arise and it would seem that this approach has been surpassed by the results obtained using the inflatable devices, particularly of Rosen and Soctt.

The external electronic stimulators, such as the anal plug electrode and the vaginal tampon electrode, have not proved successful.

Mechanical Devices

The simple use of a vaginal tampon can be of help to some women with mild stress incontinence. Devices, such as the Bonnar inflatable device and the Edwards[32] pubo-vaginal spring, have had disappointing results (see Chapter 9).

The Incontinence Nurse Adviser

The appointment of an incontinence nurse adviser in our urological department has proved to be an extremely successful measure. A nurse adviser undertakes home visits to assess not only the patient, but also the problem and the particular environmental factors. She arranges for the patient to attend the hospital for further investigation, or, if necessary, to be admitted on a short-stay basis for further evaluation. Her role in communicating between hospital and community has bridged a major gap that previously existed. Community nurses now attend the hospital to discuss problems which they experience with incontinent patients and the nurse adviser is able to update them on the available aids and services for their patients. Adequate supervision is essential for patients who are treated by indwelling catheters and a growing number of patients are treated by intermittent self-catheterisation. Such patients do need to be able to obtain advice at short notice.

Finally, the incontinence nurse adviser is able to undertake market research on the many appliances and garments which are now becoming available. It is important that these aids are carefully assessed for the benefit not only of the patient but also of the manufacturers.

Acknowledgment

Work on incontinence in the Clinical Research Unit, Ham Green Hospital, Bristol, is being supported by the Medical Research Council (Grant no. 974/135).

Notes

1. Wolin, L.H. (1969), 'Stress Incontinence in Young, Healthy Nulliparous Female Subjects', *J. Urol., 101*, 545-9.

2. Nemir, A. and Middleton, R.P. (1954), 'Stress Incontinence in Young Nulliparous Women: A Statistical Study', *Amer. J. Obst. & Gynec., 68*, 1166-8.

3. Thomas, T.M., Plymat, K.R., Blannin, J. and Meade, T.W. (1978), 'The Prevalence of Incontinence in The Community', paper presented at VIIIth ICS meeting, Manchester.

4. Exton-Smith, A.N., Norton, D. and McLaren, R. (1962), *An Investigation of Geriatric Nursing Problems in Hospital* (National Corporation for the Care of Old People, London).

5. Feneley, R.C.L., Shepherd, A.M., Powell, P.H. and Blannin, J. (1979), 'Urinary Incontinence in Perspective', communication to BAUS.

6. Whiteside, G. (1979), 'Symptoms of Micturition Disorders in Relation to Dynamic Function', *Urol. Clin. North America, 6*, 55-62.

7. Rankin, J.T. (1969), 'Urological Complications of Rectal Surgery', *Brit. J. Urol., 41*, 655-9.

8. Santoro, J. and Kaye, D. (1978), 'Recurrent Urinary Tract Infections: Pathogenesis and Management', *Med. Clin. North America, 62(5)*, 1005-20.

9. Frewen, W.K. (1978), 'An Objective Assessment of the Unstable Bladder of Psychosomatic Origin', *Brit. J. Urol., 50*, 246-9.

10. Stanton, S.L. (1973), 'A Comparison of Emepronium Bromide and Flavoxate Hydrocholoride in the Treatment of Urinary Incontinence', *J. Urol., 110*, 529-32.

11. Scott, M.B. and Morrow, J.W. (1978), 'Phenoxybenzamine in Neurogenic Bladder Dysfunction after Spinal Cord Injury. 1. Voiding Dysfunction', *J. Urol., 119*, 480-2.

12. Kegel, A.H. (1951), 'Physiologic Therapy for Urinary Stress Incontinence', *J.A.M.A., 146*, 915-17.

13. Hoffman, J.W. and Sokol, J.K. (1952), 'The Management of Stress Incontinence', *Geriatrics, 7*, 225-31.

14. Jones, E.G. (1965), 'Non-operative Treatment of Stress Incontinence', *Clin. Obstet. & Gynec., 6*, 220-35.

15. Moore, T. and Schofield, P.F. (1967), 'Treatment of Stress Incontinence by Maximum Perineal Electrical Stimulation', *Brit. Med. J., 3*, 150-1.

16. Collins, C.D. (1972), personal communication.

17. Shepherd, A.M. (1977), personal communication.

18. Abrams, P. and Feneley, R.C.L. (1978), 'Significance of Symptoms Associated with Bladder Outflow Obstruction', *Urol. Int., 33*, 171-4.

19. Dunn, M., Smith, J.C. and Ardran, G.M. (1974), 'Prolonged Bladder Distension as a Treatment of Urgency and Urge Incontinence of Urine', *Brit. J. Urol., 46*, 645-52.

20. Godec, C., Cass, A.S. and Ayala, G.F. (1975), 'Bladder Inhibition with Functional Electrical Stimulation', *Urology, 6(6)*, 663-6.

21. Essenhigh, D.M. and Yeates, W.K. (1973), 'Transection of the Bladder with Particular Reference to Enuresis', *Brit. J. Urol., 45*, 299-305.

22. Torrens, M.J. and Griffith, H.B. (1974), 'The Control of the Uninhibited Bladder by Selective Sacral Neurectomy', *Brit. J. Urol., 46*, 639-44.

23. Cardozo, L.D., Abrams, P.H., Stanton, S.L. and Feneley, R.C.L. (1978), 'Idiopathic Bladder Instability Treated by Bio-feedback', *Brit. J. Urol., 50*, 521-3.

24. Desmond, A.D. and Shuttleworth, K.E.D. (1977), 'The Results of Urinary Diversion in Multiple Sclerosis', *Brit. J. Urol., 49*, 495-502.

25. Morrow, J.W. and Bogaard, T.P. (1977), 'Bladder Rehabilitation in Patients with Old Spinal Cord Injuries with Bladder Neck Incision and External Sphincterotomy', *J. Urol., 117*, 164-7.

26. Lapides, J., Diokno, A.C., Silber, S.J. and Rowe, B.S. (1972), 'Clean Intermittent Self-catheterisation in the Treatment of Urinary Tract Disease', *J. Urol., 107*, 458-61.

27. Withycombe, J., Whitaker, R. and Hunt, G. (1978), 'Intermittent Catheterisation in the Management of Children with Neuropathic Bladder', *Lancet, 2(8097)*, 981-3.

28. Kaufman, J.J. (1973), 'Urethral Compression for the Treatment of Post-prostatectomy Incontinence', *J. Urol., 110*, 93-6.

29. Scott, F.B., Bradley, W.E. and Timm, G.W. (1974), 'Treatment of Urinary Incontinence by an Implantable Prosthetic Urinary Sphincter', *J. Urol., 112*, 75-80.

30. Rosen, M. (1976), 'A Simple Artificial Implantable Sphincter', *Brit. J. Urol., 48*, 675-80.

31. Caldwell, K.P.S. (1967), 'The Treatment of Incontinence by Electronic Implants', *Ann. Roy. Coll. Surg., 41*, 447-59.

32. Edwards, L. (1971), 'The Control of Incontinence of Urine in Women with a Pubo-vaginal Spring Device: Objective and Subjective Results', *Brit. J. Urol.*, *43*, 211-25.

3 GYNAECOLOGICAL ASPECTS

Stuart L. Stanton

By tradition lower urinary tract disorders in the female have been managed by the gynaecologist, but with the development of the speciality of urology, they have received increased attention from the urologist. The benefits of his special knowledge of the pathophysiology of the urethra and bladder must be seen in the context of the gynaecologist's familiarity with the adjacent female genital tract and the frequent close association between its diseases and those of the lower urinary tract. Thus the argument as to which speciality is better qualified to treat these disorders in women cannot readily be answered. Rather, the patîent is likely to obtain greater benfit from the close co-operation between urologist and gynaecologist if she is managed by whichever clinician has a specialised interest and experience in this subject.

The following terms need to be defined:

Stress incontinence is a symptom or a sign meaning loss of urine on exertion, without active bladder contraction. It may imply that urethral sphincter incompetence is present (see Chapter 1, p. 30).

Urge incontinence is the involuntary loss of urine associated with a strong desire to void. This may be accompanied by a detrusor contraction (see Chapter 1, p. 31).

Frequency is the passage of urine seven or more times during the day or the need to wake more than twice at night to void.

Classification of Incontinence

A more scientific approach to the management of incontinence during the last two decades has resulted in an improved prognosis for patients with this condition and accurate diagnosis remains an important first step in their management. The classification of the causes of incontinence as found in a consecutive series of 362 patients seen in our urodynamic unit are shown with their incidence in Table 3.1.[1]

The most common causes of urinary incontinence in younger and middle aged women are:

(1) Urethral sphincter incompetence, which presents with stress incontinence and additional symptoms sometimes of urgency, urge

Table 3.1: Causes of Incontinence in 362 Patients

Causes	Percentage
Urethral sphincter incompetence	49.9
Detrusor instability	38.5
Overflow incontinence	1.9
Fistulae	1.1
Congenital	0.3
Functional	8.6

incontinence and frequency. There may be associated genital prolapse with backache and 'a dropping feeling' experienced in the vulvoperineal region.

(2)   Detrusor instability, more common in the elderly than urethral sphincter incompetence, as the former can be secondary to cerebral atherosclerosis: otherwise it may be secondary to an upper motor neurone lesion, previous bladder neck surgery or psychosomatic disorder, the latter implying a loss of the normal cortical inhibition of the detrusor muscle. Implicit in the causation of incontinence associated with detrusor instability, is a degree of incompetence of the urethral sphincter mechanism, which permits escape of urine as the detrusor contracts uninhibitedly. In some cases of detrusor instability, no cause can be found. The main symptoms are urge incontinence, frequency and stress incontinence, and neurological symptoms are present when a neuropathic aetiology exists.

(3)   Retention with overflow may present with continuous or stress incontinence, and frequency. Upper renal tract dilatation may accompany this with symptoms of loin pain and sometimes superadded urinary tract infection.

(4)   Congenital disorders such as ectopic ureter and epispadias may demonstrate continuous incontinence or stress incontinence respectively.

(5)   Fistulae between the bladder or ureter, and the vagina will cause continuous incontinence. Proximal urethral fistulae may cause stress incontinence or continuous incontinence, depending upon whether the fistula has rendered the sphincter mechanism incompetent, whilst distal urethral fistulae may be asymptomatic.

(6)   Finally, functional causes should not be omitted. In some patients, it may be impossible to demonstrate any abnormality, and the diagnosis is made by the exclusion of an obvious cause and by the clinician's high index of suspicion that the patient has psychiatric rather than organic pathology.

Gynaecological Conditions Affecting the Bladder and Urethral Function

The close developmental origin and anatomical proximity of the genital and lower urinary tracts means that pathological processes affecting one may commonly affect the other as well.

The urological symptoms complained of by women include incontinence, frequency, urgency and urge incontinence, dysuria (pain on voiding), difficulty in voiding and slow stream. Symptoms are rarely single but are usually combined, e.g. urgency and frequency. They may also be combined with gynaecological symptoms such as prolapse or vaginal menstrual cycle. The second half of the cycle is progesterone-dominated which leads to a worsening of symptoms of stress incontinence prior to the period as it has a relaxant effect on smooth muscle and ligamentous supports. Some women admit to increased frequency of micturition at period time.

Pregnancy

Frequency usually starts in the first trimester and worsens as pregnancy progresses. This is partly due to increased fluid intake in early pregnancy and in part to the mechanical effects of the enlarging uterus.[2, 3] Stress incontinence occurs in 53 per cent of primigravida and 85 per cent of multigravidae during pregnancy, with 42 per cent of patients complaining of this symptom before pregnancy.[4] Its onset in the three trimesters appears similar and according to Francis, if it has not been experienced in the pregnancy under review or in the puerperium following a previous pregnancy it is not likely to occur. Voiding difficulties and retention may occur around 14 weeks due to impaction of a retroverted gravid uterus, following a difficult labour with vaginal bruising, or associated with neglected aftercare of an epidural anaesthetic.

Menopause

The effects of increasing oestrogen deficiency at the time of the menopause are noticed on the bladder and urethra as well as on the genital tissues. This leads to symptoms of incontinence (as bladder neck supports weaken and the hermetic closure of the urethral mucosa is less effective), urgency and frequency, and the urethral syndrome (frequency and dysuria). Osborne[5] studied the symptom of frequency in a broad age spectrum in a group of 600 women and found an increase in nocturia over the age of 50 years, but no change of the incidence of diurnal frequency with age. There are, however, additional factors to be considered, namely the role of anxiety and other psychological disturbances encountered at the menopause which can affect bladder function.

Pelvic Mass

Frequency of micturition and occasional urgency can be produced by a pelvic mass such as a gravid uterus, a fibroid or an ovarian cyst. A large pelvic mass and a retrogravid uterus can produce retention with overflow incontinence. Rarely, ureteric obstruction may occur.

Endometriosis

This condition may affect the bladder and ureters. Urethral involvement is, however, rare.[6] Symptoms are usually worse prior to and during menstruation and include dysuria frequency and urgency. Cyclical haematuria may be encountered.

Congenital Malformations

These include hydrocolpos, haematocolpos and epispadias. Hydrocolpos, a collection of watery fluid which accumulates behind a membrane in the region of the hymen, is encountered in the first few days of life and may lead to urinary infection. Haematocolpos may present at puberty with a history of monthly abdominal pain, an abdominal swelling, difficulty in micturition or retention and amenorrhoea. In both conditions incision of the membrane under sterile conditions and drainage is curative. Epispadias may not be detected until adult life and results from failure of fusion of midline mesodermal structures leading to a short and wide bladder neck with poor sphincteric musculature and stress incontinence (see Figure 3.1).

Prolapse

Anterior vaginal wall prolapse may either take the form of a cystocoele, where the base of the bladder descends, or a cystourethrocoele where in addition there is descent of the proximal urethra and bladder neck. With the former, stress incontinence is not so likely as the bladder neck is elevated, but urgency and frequency may occur especially if there is a residual urine which has become infected. A cystourethrocoele may cause symptoms of stress incontinence, urgency and frequency. Ureteric compression leading to hydroureter and hydronephrosis can occur where there is concomitant uterine prolapse.

Pelvic Malignancy

Spread of malignancy from the ovary, body of the uterus or cervix can

Figure 3.1: Female Epispadias

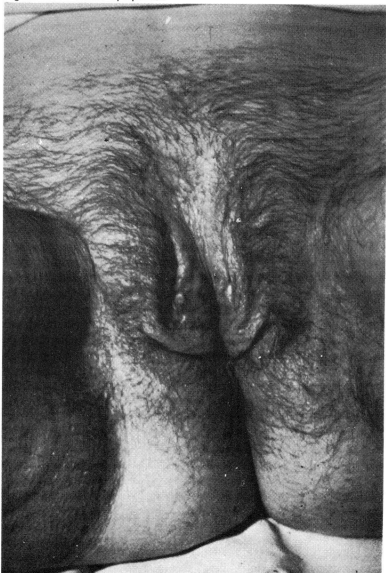

Source: Reproduced with kind permission from Stanton, S.L. (1974), 'Gynecologic Complications of Epispadias and Bladder Exstrophy', *American Journal of
Obstetrics and Gynecology, 119*, 749-54.

lead to ureteric compression and uraemia. Direct invasion of the bladder can lead to vesical fistula. Primary or secondary vaginal carcinomas can invade the bladder producing a vesico-vagina fistula, although both are uncommon. Finally, fistulae can follow surgical or radiotherapeutic treatment of pelvic carcinoma.

Post-Wertheim's or Radical Pelvic Surgery

In the course of a Wertheim's operation or other radical pelvic surgery to control pelvic malignancy, the autonomic nerve fibres to the bladder are often cut. This results in a hypotonic bladder which can become overdistended if the bladder is inadequately drained post-operatively.

Pelvic Inflammatory Disease

Infection of the genital tract may simultaneously occur with infection of the lower urinary tract, leading to symptoms of abdominal pain, a purulent vaginal discharge, dysuria and frequency. Extensive pelvic inflammatory disease may cause dilatation of the upper urinary tract with delayed urinary drainage which may resolve following adequate medical or surgical treatment.

Urinary Fistulae

Fistulae may occur between the urethra, bladder or ureter and the vagina. In the developed countries the most frequent causes are gynaecological and include surgical trauma to the ureters and bladder at hysterectomy, neoplastic involvement of bladder and urethera and as a sequel to pelvic irradiation in the treatment of neoplasm. In countries with restricted maternity services, obstetric injuries are more common, particularly pressure necrosis of the bladder following prolonged cephalo-pelvic disproportion in labour and leading to a vesico-vaginal fistula.

The Patient

Urinary incontinence may affect women at any age. Apart from congenital lesions, Nemir and Middleton[7] found that five per cent of young nulliparous women had troublesome stress incontinence. At the other extreme, Isaacs and Walkey[8] record an incidence of 46 per cent in long-stay geriatric female patients. Between the ages of 20 and 60, incontinence due to urethral sphincter incompetence is commonest, whilst after 60 the proportion of patients with detrusor instability due to cerebro-vascular atherosclerosis gradually rises.

Patients with incontinence are usually socially very conscious of their disability and may be too ashamed to seek medical advice and in extreme cases, will become social recluses. Occasionally they have been ill-advised and told that nothing can be done for them. Apathy and lack of interest are still encountered among some medical and nursing staff and a lack of awareness of modern concepts in the management of incontinence is still a frequent occurrence.

The effect of incontinence on the patient and her relatives is not hard to imagine. The patient becomes limited in her activities and independence. If she has urge incontinence, she never knows when a sudden desire to urinate will precipitate uncontrolled leakage. She develops frequency in an attempt to minimise the urine loss by keeping her bladder as empty as possible, so that she is in constant search of toilet facilities. The winter months are worst to endure because cold aggravates frequency and coughs are more prevalent. Sports are abandoned because the physical effort precipitates incontinence and she may be afraid to sit down in public because she will wet the chair. Black is a favourite colour to wear as it discolours least and often diguises urinary leakage.

The relatives, but not always the patient, are readily aware of the urinary odour and tact has to be exercised by all. Very often urinary leakage is the final reason to despatch the elderly relative to institutional care, yet all too frequently this is one reason which institutions for the elderly use to debar such people (see Chapters 11 and 13). For older people, incontinence means loss of independence and sometimes separation from their families, a hard price to pay when good medical and nursing care can do so much to remedy this. To accept incontinence in the elderly in the absence of dementia as a natural outcome of growing old is a step backwards into nineteenth century medicine.

Some patients have psychological disorders which require additional investigation and treatment. Hafner *et al.*[9] showed that in the absence of organic bladder or urethral abnormality, symptoms of urgency and urge incontinence have a treatable neurotic aetiology in 50 per cent of women. Patients with a low neurotic score on psychiatric assessment responded poorly to therapy as they denied or disclaimed their symptoms and so were resistant to treatment.

Criteria for Referral to a Gynaecologist

It is still a common finding that patients will endure incontinence for many years before seeking medical advice. Once seen by their primary care physician there is little to be gained by delay in referral to a specialist. Apart from testing the urine to detect a urinary tract infection and confirming that the patient wishes to have her incontinence treated, she should be referred for specialist management. Although many patients can respond satisfactorily to physiotherapy exercises, it is as well to ensure that the cause of incontinence does not require prior surgical or medical treatment (see Chapters 2 and 9).

Patients with the following symptom complexes are usually referred to the gynaecologist – stress incontinence with or without urgency and frequency, recurrent stress incontinence, and stress incontinence with prolapse.

About ten per cent of new patients attending a gynaecologist may have a primary complaint of incontinence. Children and the elderly with incontinence are usually referred to the paediatrician and geriatrician respectively. Patients with symptoms of urinary tract infection, haematuria or difficulty in voiding are conventionally referred to the urologist. Should there be dominant neurological symptoms the patient may be referred to a neurologist. Thus although the gynaecologist may see the greater proportion of women who complain of incontinence, many other specialities become involved in their care.

Role of the Urodynamic Unit

A urodynamic unit offers a specialised interest and experience in the management of disorders and micturition and of the lower urinary tract. The unit may either be directed by a urologist or a gynaecologist, the former looking after both male and female patients whilst the latter usually investigates only the female (see Chapter 2). Because of the capital costs of equipment and need for highly trained staff these units are at present usually organised on a Regional rather than an Area basis. Their future development will depend partly upon patient demand and partly on the finances available. The advantage, like in any specialised unit, lies in the the total experience gained from a wide variety of patients referred to it and in turn in the extensive variety of surgical, medical and 'mechanical' forms of treatment (e.g. incontinence pads and garments and devices) which it can offer its patients (see Chapter 9).

The unit is advantageously placed to carry out ethically approved research (with patient consent) which forms the basis of future investigations and treatment, and finally it can offer unique teaching experience to medical and nursing staff and to medical students.

Investigations

Lower urinary tract investigations have been discussed in Chapters 1 and 2. Here I shall consider the clinical history and examination oriented towards the gynaecological patient, and the investigation of videocystourethrography, which is the combination of cystometry and radiological screening of the bladder.

History and Examination

The history should cover the main gynaecological symptoms including the menstrual cycle, contraception, pelvic pain, prolapse and vaginal discharge. The first part of a questionnaire used at the Urodynamic Unit, St George's Hospital, London is shown in Figure 3.2. Neurological questions include weakness of limbs, rectal soiling and the presence of backache. A note of any psychiatric disorder and the current and past drug history are important. Past history includes an obstetric record and note of pelvic operations – particularly those likely to have involved the bladder and urethra. The clinical examination must include a neurological and pelvic examination. Incontinence is best examined by asking the patient to cough whilst standing in the erect position.

Videocystourethrography

There are many different approaches to the investigation of bladder disorders. They depend on a variety of factors including an understanding of the mechanism of continence and incontinence and the finances and technical resources available.

We have used videocystourethrography (VCU) as our standard investigation for the last five years[10] (see Figure 3.3). This technique was developed in San Francisco by Enhorning, Miller and Hinman (Jnr)[11] in 1964 and first used in England at the Middlesex Hospital by Bates and Whiteside.[12] Although all our patients are investigated by this method, I would recommend that, where this service is restricted, it could be limited to those patients who have a complicated history with mixed symptomatology and those patients who have had one unsuccessful operation for incontinence.

Figure 3.2: The First Part of the Urodynamic Questionnaire Used at the Urodynamic Unit, St George's Hospital, London

ST. GEORGE'S HOSPITAL

Card No. 1

URODYNAMIC DATA 1

Surname   Hosp. No _____   2 5

Unit No .... (2.5)

Ref. Consultant ....   First Names   (10 15) Date of Birth   6 9

Date of Consultation .... (6.9)   Sex

PRESENT CONDITION   (9   No Data)   Age 10 15

Main Complaints   Duration

1)   16 18

2)   19 21

3)   22 24

Duration: 0 < $\frac{1}{12}$ 1 = $\frac{1.6}{12}$ 2 = $\frac{7.12}{12}$ 3 = $\frac{13}{12}$ 2yrs. 4 = 3-5yrs. 5 = 5-10yrs. 6 = >10yrs.

Frequency Day < Hourly   0=No, 1= $\{\frac{9.1}{10}\}$ 2= $\{\frac{2}{7.9}\}$ 3= $\{\frac{3}{5.6}\}$ 4= $\{\frac{4}{4}\}$ 5= $\{\frac{5}{3.4}\}$ 6= $\{\frac{6}{3}\}$ 7= $\{\frac{7}{2.3}\}$ 8= $\{\frac{8}{2}\}$ 25   26

Night: No. of times: 0 = None, 1 2 3 4 5 6 7 8+ 9 = No Data

Other Symptoms   0=No   1=Yes occasionally 2=Yes frequently   3=Not applicable

Stress Incontinence (27)	Urgency (28)	27 28
Urgency Incontinence (29)	Wet at rest (30)	29 30
Wet on standing up (31)	Wet at night (32)	31 32
Ability to interrupt flow (33)	Complete emptying (34)	33 34
Post micturition dribble (35)	Good stream (36)	35 36
Straining to void (37)	Retention of urine (38)	37 38
Dysuria (39)	Aware of full bladder (40)	39 40
Aware of being wet (41)	Aware of prolapse dragging (42)	41 42
Protective underwear (43)	Dyspareunia (44)	43 44
Rectal soiling (45)	Weakness of legs (46)	45 46
Cough (47)	Constipation (48)	47 48
Other symptoms 1)		49 50
2)		51 52

Periods   1 = Premen., 2 = Menopausal, 3 = Postmen., 4 = Hysterectomy +/BSO   53
             O.C.Pill ....   Cycle ....   LMP

Effect of a period on a main symptom   0 = No Effect   2 = Aggravated   3 = Better   54
                                            9 = No Data or No periods

Diabetes Mellitus   0 = No 1 = Yes 9 = No Data   55

Neurological disorder 0 = None 1 = UMN lesion 2 = LMN lesion 3 = Mixed 4 = Unspecified   56
                           5 = MS 9 = No Data

Psychological disorder   0 = None 1 = Schizophrenia 2 = Other Psychosis 3 = Neurosis   57

Other Disorders 1)   58 59
                     2)   60 61

Present Medication   Name   Success   Duration

1)   62 66

2)   67 71

3)   72 76

Success: 0 = No success   1 = Improved 2 = Cured   3 = Irrelevant 9 = No Data

Other   1)   77 78

           2)   79 80

Figure 3.3: Schema for Videocystourethrography

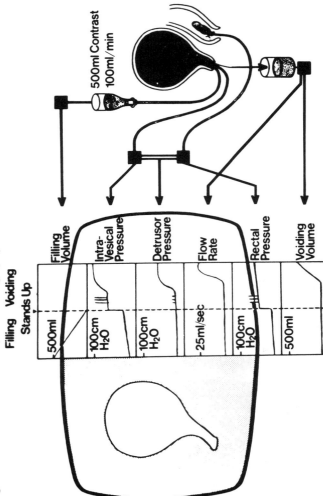

Simultaneous recording of the bladder and rectal pressure changes during supine cystometry, combined with a display of bladder filling volume is shown on the left hand side of the polygraph trace. On voiding, the bladder and rectal pressures together with the voiding rate and volume are recorded on the right of the trace. A television camera selects three parameters (intravesical pressure, detrusor pressure and voiding rate) which are added to the radiographic image of the bladder (shown on the extreme left of the scheme) and recorded with sound commentary on the video-tape.

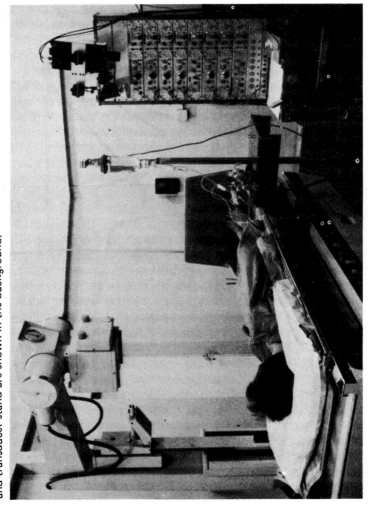

Figure 3.4: Patient and Radiographic Tipping Table. The recorder with the television camera and transducer stand are shown in the background.

After the procedure has been explained to the patient, she lies flat on the radiological table and her bladder is filled in a sterile fashion with contrast media (see Figure 3.4). Fine pressure recording catheters are placed in the bladder and rectum. She is asked to say when first sensation and full bladder capacity are reached. Filling of the bladder then ceases and the filling catheter is removed. She is brought to the upright position on the tipping table and radiologically screened in the oblique erect position. This allows good visualisation of the bladder neck and base of the bladder. She is asked to cough several times to check competence of the sphincter mechanism and then allowed to void, the contrast medium being collected in a uroflowmeter. She is asked to interrupt micturition after approximately 200-250 ml have been voided, in order to test the ability of the sphincter mechanism to close and to effect milk-back of urine into the bladder. Voiding is then continued to completion and any residue is recorded. The total time for the study is about 20 minutes.

During the investigation there is continuous recording of bladder pressures and during voiding the urine flow rate and volume voided are also recorded, so that the pressure in the bladder can always be related to the volume of fluid it contains and *vice versa*.

The final picture on the monitor consists of the radiological image and simultaneous bladder pressure and urine flow recordings. These are recorded together with sound commentary on video-tape, for future replay. A normal recording of the filling and voiding phases is shown in Figure 3.5 and a video-image demonstrating stress incontinence due to urethral sphincter incompetence is demonstrated in Figure 3.6.

The advantages of VCU are:

(1)   it is an informative, reproducible and consistent investigation;
(2)   normal and abnormal urethra and bladder function can be demonstrated; and
(3)   changes in the anatomical support of the bladder neck and base of bladder are easily visualised.

The disadvantages are:

(1)   the cost of equipment, which is approximately £12,000, excluding radiological equipment;
(2)   a radiologist, nurse and technician are required; and
(3)   the dose of irradiation to the ovaries is approximately 700 mr/min which is less than that of an intravenous urogram series.

Figure 3.5: A Normal Trace Showing Filling and Voiding Phases with Multiple Voluntary Interruptions of Voiding

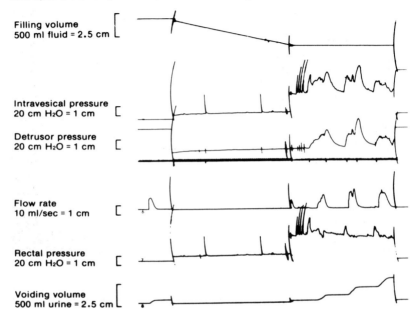

Filling volume
500 ml fluid = 2.5 cm

Intravesical pressure
20 cm H₂O = 1 cm

Detrusor pressure
20 cm H₂O = 1 cm

Flow rate
10 ml/sec = 1 cm

Rectal pressure
20 cm H₂O = 1 cm

Voiding volume
500 ml urine = 2.5 cm

Urilos

With some patients it is not possible to confirm the history by detecting 'urine' loss at VCU or when objective evidence of the result of a surgical procedure to cure incontinence is sought, it may be impractical to repeat the VCU. A non-invasive test to overcome this difficulty, has been designed by James.[13] It involves wearing a disposable paper nappy containing aluminium strip electrodes and dry electrolyte (see Figure 3.7). The patient attends for the test with a comfortably full bladder, wears the nappy under her pants adjacent to her vulva and over a period of 45 minutes she exercises, drinks and simulates her normal day-to-day activities which might ordinarily precipitate urine loss at home. Any urinary leakage is detected by a recorder attached to the nappy.[14]

Figure 3.6: The Final Video-image Showing Stress Incontinence Due to Urethral Sphincter Incompetence

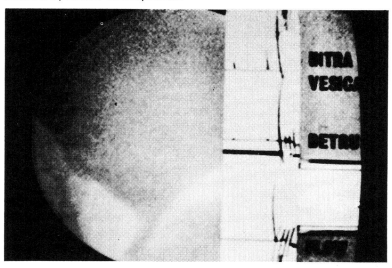

Figure 3.7: The Urilos Monitor, Single-channel Recorder and Disposable Electronic Nappy

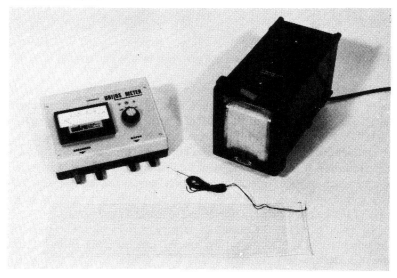

Treatment

The treatment of incontinence is dependent upon its cause. Therefore whilst indicating broad guidelines it should be remembered that individual patients may require minor modifications or a combination of therapy rather than a single method.

Role of Surgery

Urethral Sphincter Incompetence. The principal indication for surgery is urethral sphincter incompetence. The surgical aims are to elevate the bladder neck and raise bladder neck resistance. Any anterior vaginal wall prolapse can be corrected simultaneously.

The two main surgical approaches are vaginal (anterior repair or colporrhaphy) and suprapubic. The former is conventional but lacks the effective sustained cure rate of the suprapubic operations (e.g. Marshall-Marchetti-Krantz operation, the Burch colposuspension and sling procedures). These are carried out via an abdominal incision (a sling procedure will also require a vaginal incision) and are more major procedures than an anterior repair. The operation is usually followed by a brief period of catheter drainage and a stay in hospital of seven to ten days. Cure rates for vaginal repair vary from 35 to 75 per cent. My preference is a modification of the Burch colposuspension operation in which I insert additional sutures alongside the bladder base between the paravaginal fascia and ileo-pectineal ligaments. This provides additional support for the anterior vaginal wall. This is the only suprapubic procedure which will effectively correct anterior vaginal wall prolapse as well as incontinence. At a two year follow-up, our overall cure rate for incontinence was 86 per cent.[15]

Whichever operation is chosen, there are some simple post-operative rules. Heavy lifting is to be permanently eschewed: incontinence surgery is only as good as the patient's tissues, regardless of the suture material. A gradual return to normal activity within three months is recommended. If childbearing is not complete, the operation should be deferred until it is, as a subsequent vaginal delivery is likely to produce a recurrence of incontinence. Intercourse should not be resumed until two months after surgery to allow healing to be complete and in the case of the colposuspension operation, to avoid dyspareunia.

In order to assess the results of surgery, a follow-up with objective documentation is necessary. We review our patients three to four months after surgery for clinical and VCU assessment and then yearly for a clinical assessment and Urilos test.

Detrusor Instability. Where detrusor instability is responsible for incontinence, surgery should be postponed until drug therapy has been tried. Surgery can be used to correct any associated urethral sphincter incompetence however occasionally this may make detrusor instability worse. Two main techniques have evolved for the specific treatment of instability. These are sacral nerve root denervation (S2, 3 and 4) and vaginal denervation (inferior hypogastric plexus). They produce about a 50 per cent improvement and are not commonly performed (see also Chapter 2, p. 50).

Retention with Overflow. Retention with overflow may be helped by a urethrotomy which enlarges the lumen of the urethra by a series of evenly spaced longitudinal incisions. If retention is not relieved, progressive difficulty in voiding with upper tract dilatation and superadded urinary tract infection may occur, leading to deterioration of renal function. A urological opinion should be sought at an early stage as a urinary diversion may be required (see also Chapter 2, p. 50).

Drugs

Drugs are used in two situations: to control incontinence (by increasing urethral resistance, or diminishing uninhibited detrusor activity); and to overcome retention with overflow (by stimulating the detrusor to empty effectively, or lowering urethral resistance) (see also Chapter 2, p. 42).

Incontinence. The urethra and bladder neck are rich in alpha-adrenergic receptors and drugs which stimulate them will increase urethral resistance, e.g. phenylpropanolamine (5mg t.d.s.).

There are a variety of drugs which diminish uninhibited detrusor activity. They include anticholinergic agents (probanthine 10-15 mg t.d.s. imipramine (Tofranil) 25-50 mg bd or nocte), ganglion-blocking agents (emepronium bromide (Cetiprin) 200 mg q.d.s. – taken with water to reduce the risk of mucosal ulceration) and musculotrophic agents (flavoxate hydrochloride (Urispas) 200 mg q.d.s.) All of them produce about a 50 per cent improvement in symptoms. Newer drugs include prostaglandin-synthetase inhibitors (indomethacin (Indocid) 50 mg t.d.s. or q.d.s.; flurbiprofen (Froben) 50 mg tds.).[16,17] These have been shown to decrease symptoms in up to 85 per cent of patients.

Retention with Overflow. Cholinergic preparations (carbachol 2 mg q.d.s., bethanechol (Myotonine) 5 mg t.d.s. whilst stimulating the detrusor to contract may also increase urethral resistance, so there may be no improvement. Urethral resistance may be diminished by the use of alpha-blocking agents (phenoxybenzamine 10 mg in increasing dosage until side-effects occur).

Functional Conditions

Anxiety, depression and other psychiatric states can produce urological symptoms[9] and can cause detrusor instability. Psychiatric referral for diagnosis and treatment is of benefit.

Role of Bladder Drill and Bio-feedback

Where detrusor instability is secondary to psychosomatic disorder, control by bladder drill[18] or bio-feedback[19] have been shown to be effective. Frewen, to whom we owe much for the management of this condition, suggests an inpatient stay of ten days during which time the patient is taught about her condition and how to overcome her symptoms. A micturition chart helps her to prolong the intervals between voiding and adjunct therapy with 10 mg of diazepam is employed: an 82 per cent cure has been achieved. Bio-feedback using auditory and visual stimuli obtained from the abnormal increase in bladder pressure, trains the patient to regain bladder control. Fine pressure-measuring catheters are inserted into the bladder and rectum, and cystometry is performed to elicit uninhibited contractions. The patient attends for hourly sessions once a week for six to eight weeks, when she is taught methods of muscle relaxation. Between sessions she keeps a urinary diary to measure symptomatic improvement. About 80 per cent of patients are helped by this.

Role of Physiotherapy

It would seem that physiotherapy is indicated as adjuvant therapy in the absence of gross anatomical damage and following corrective surgery for incontinence where symptoms persist and where there is laxity of the pelvic floor musculature. It would be helpful to evaluate these exercises in order to define precisely their contribution and to devise new techniques in the light of increased knowledge of the anatomy and physiology of this region (see Chapter 10 and Appendix to it).

Validation of Treatment

In order to determine the true rather than the panacea effect, each mode of treatment should be evaluated objectively and subjectively.

In the case of surgery, a follow-up time of at least two and preferably five years is required to determine cure and any long-term side effects. Drug studies should be controlled, double-blinded and randomised. Evaluation of pads and garments requires subjective as well as objective laboratory investigation to determine the physical properties of pads and their behaviour under varying conditions.

Role of the Specialist Nurse

Although the role of the incontinence nurse adviser is referred to in Chapter 9, it is relevant to consider her position in a urodynamic unit. I would understand her to have four main duties.

Investigation. She would be responsible for the care of the patient during investigation which involves explanation of the procedure and reassurance. In our unit the nurse carries out many of the investigations including catheterisation for cystometry, cystometry and urethral pressure profile measurements, with the doctor present for the interpretation of the results.

Incontinence Aids. We have a 'pads and garments advisory service', organised and maintained by the nurse, where patients are advised on the most appropriate choice. The service is available in the hospital and for a trial period within the community. The nurse helps the patient obtain the pads and advises the community nurses and health visitors on which are available (see Chapter 9).

Teaching. In order to integrate the care of the incontinent patient and the work of the unit with the hospital and community, the nurse serves a vital role by teaching student nurses and advising nursing colleagues on the wards and in the community, and by speaking to lay groups within the community. Some of these groups, notably the Multiple Sclerosis Societies are usually extremely well informed and any lecture given to them is often as technical as those given to colleagues.

Research. Not all nurses wish to carry out research. However, a specialised nursing position often carries an option to become involved in clinical nursing research sometimes leading to a higher degree.

Summary

The management of incontinence can be complicated and requires the involvement of medical, nursing and biomedical disciplines. Over the last ten years many advances in investigation have taken place. The priorities are now for research into non-invasive techniques of investigation, the management of incontinence in the elderly and the drug control of uninhibited bladder contractions. Just how much progress is achieved will depend upon the importance attached by the community and medical and nursing professions to the disabling effects of incontinence.

Notes

1.   Cardozo, L. (1979), 'Use of Flurbiprofen in the Management of Detrusor Instability', unpublished MD thesis, University of Liverpool, Chapter 2.

2.   Francis, W. (1960), 'Disturbances of Bladder Function in Relation to Pregnancy', *J. Obstet. & Gynaec. Brit. Emp.*, *67*, 353-66.

3.   Parboosingh, J. and Doig, A. (1973), 'Studies of Nocturia in Normal Pregnancy', *J. Obstet. & Gynaec. Brit. Comm.*, *80*, 888-95.

4.   Francis, W. (1960), 'Onset of Stress Incontinence', *J. Obstet. & Gynaec. Brit. Emp.*, *67*, 899-903.

5.   Osborne, J. (1976), 'Post-menopausal Changes in Micturition Habits and Urine Flow and Urethral Pressure Studies' in Campbell, S. (ed.), *Management of Menopause and Post-menopausal Years* (MTP, Lancaster), 285-9.

6.   Lifschitz, S. and Buchsbaum, H. (1978), 'Urinary Tract Involvement by Benign and Malignant Gynecologic Disease' in Buchsbaum, H. and Schmidt, J.D. (eds.), *Gynecologic and Obstetric Urology* (W.B. Saunders, Philadelphia), 359-72.

7.   Nemir, A. and Middleton, R. (1954), 'Stress Incontinence in Young Nulliparous Women', *Amer. J. Obstet. & Gynec.*, *68*, 1166-8.

8.   Isaacs, B. and Walkey, F. (1964), 'A Survey of Incontinence in Elderly Hospital Patients', *Geront. Clin.*, *6*, 367-76.

9.   Hafner, R.J., Stanton, S. and Guy, J. (1977), 'Psychiatric Study of Women with Urgency and Urge Incontinence', *Brit. J. Urol.*, *49*, 211-14.

10.   Stanton, S.L. (1977), *Female Urinary Incontinence* (Lloyd-Luke, London), 45-8.

11.   Enhorning, G., Miller, E. and Hinman, F. Jnr. (1964), 'Urethral Closure Studied by Cine-roentgenography and Simultaneous Bladder-urethra Pressure Recording', *Surg. Gynec. Obstet.*, *118*, 507-16.

12.   Bates, C.P., Whiteside, C.G. and Turner-Warwick, R. (1970), 'Synchronous Cine/Pressure/Flow/Cysto-urethrography with Special Reference to Stress and Urge Incontinence', *Brit. J. Urol.*, *42*, 714-23.

13.   James, E.D., Flack, F., Caldwell, K.P. and Martin, M. (1971), 'Continuous Measurement of Urine Loss and Frequency in Incontinent Patients', *Brit. J. Urol.*, *43*, 233-7.

14.   Stanton, S. and Ritchie, D. (1977), 'Urilos: A Practical Detection of Urine Loss', *Amer. J. Obstet. Gynec.*, *124*, 461-3.

15.   Stanton, S. and Cardozo, L. (1979), 'The Colposuspension Operation for Incontinence and Prolapse: Clinical Aspects', *Brit. J. Obstet. Gynaec.*, *86*, 693-7.

16. Cardozo, L. and Stanton, S. (1980), 'A Comparison between Bromo-criptine and Indomethacin in the Treatment of Detrusor Instability, *J. Urol., 123,* 399-401.

17. Cardozo, L. (1979), 'Use of Flurbiprofen in the Management of Detrusor Instability', unpublished MD thesis, University of Liverpool, Chapter 8.

18. Frewen, W.K. (1978), 'An Objective Assessment of the Unstable Bladder of Psychosomatic Origin', *Brit. J. Urol., 50,* 246-9.

19. Cardozo, L., Abrams, P., Stanton, S. and Feneley, R. (1978), 'Idiopathic Bladder Instability Treated by Bio-feedback', *Brit. J. Urol., 50,* 521-3.

FAECAL INCONTINENCE

Sir Alan G. Parks

The pathetic state of patients with incontinence is described elsewhere in this book. This chapter aims to give some description of the normal physiology of the ano-rectal region coupled with the pathophysiological changes found in patients with faecal incontinence.

Anatomy

Developmentally, the ano-rectal region is composite in structure, consisting of two tube-like components, one within the other. The inner consists of the termination of the alimentary viscus (the visceral component) and contains only smooth muscle innervated by the autonomic nervous system (Figure 4.1). The external anal sphincters form the outer structure (the somatic or skeletal muscle component), composed of skeletal muscle which is mainly under reflex control but is also influenced by conscious motivation. This component not only has a sphincteric action but its upper part (the levator-ani muscles) fans out to close the pelvic hiatus. The visceral component of the anal canal has a longitudinal layer of muscle, a circular layer (the internal sphincter), submucosa and mucosa. The internal sphincter is a fairly large muscle mass which superficially resembles the thickened segment of the circular muscle of the lower rectum. There are, however, profound functional and anatomical differences between them. The upper half of the anal canal is lined by columnar, mucus-secreting epithelium identical with that of the rectum. In the course of development, ectoderm migrates into the lower half of the anal canal which is lined by squamous epithelium as a result. The importance of this is that the squamous mucosa is dry and does not secrete mucus; it is also richly innervated with nerve endings and plays an important part in the mechanism of continence. The muco-cutaneous junction about half way along the canal is fixed to the underlying internal sphincter so that columnar epithelium cannot prolapse externally.

The somatic or skeletal muscle component of the pelvic floor is comprised of the external sphincters, the pubo-rectalis and the levator-ani muscles (pubo-coccygeus and ileo-coccygeus). The external sphincter

Figure 4.1: In this Diagrammatic Coronal Section Through the Pelvic Floor the Visceral and Somatic Components are Readily Seen, Separated by the Intersphincteric Plane

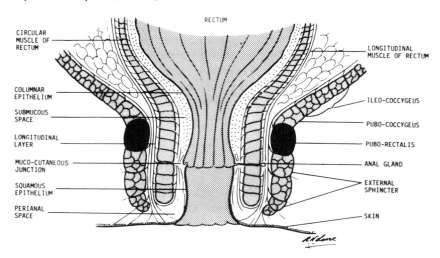

is usually divided into three parts but functionally it is a unity. Its innervation is derived from the inferior haemorrhoidal nerve. The pubo-rectalis muscle is probably the most powerful of all. It arises from the pubic ramus near the mid-line anteriorly and passes behind the upper anal canal as a sling. It therefore has a sphincteric action on all the viscera of the pelvic hiatus and at the same time has the important task of maintaining the angulation between the lower rectum and the anal canal. The levator-ani muscles have no sphincteric activity but have an anti-gravity function, preventing herniation of the visceral contents through the pelvis. Innervation of the levators and probably the pubo-rectalis comes from the branch of S4 which descends on the anterior surface of the levator muscles. The blood supply to the skeletal muscles of the pelvic floor enters via the lower and outer aspect.

In between the two components of the pelvic floor there is an embryonic plane of fusion. In the normal person very few blood vessels cross this plane and practically no nervous structures. It is of practical importance in as much as fistula tracks tend to spread within it. In addition it is a useful plane of dissection for certain operative procedures, as no important structures are encountered in it.[1]

Physiology

The Visceral Component

The importance of the squamous mucosa of the lower 2 cm of the anal canal has been mentioned. Its rich innervation gives rise to conscious sensory information.[2] If flatus or faeces enter the anal canal stimulation of the receptors causes immediate contraction of the external sphincter. The internal sphincter itself maintains closure of the anal canal in the resting state. The effective length of the sphincter can be observed by inserting a pressure probe into the lower rectum and drawing it down through the canal, recording the pressure changes *en route* (Figure 4.2). The length, about 3.5 cm, is greater in men than women by about 0.5 cm and is unrelated to age or parity. The pressure profile tends to be greater in men and diminishes with increasing age in both sexes.[3]

Figure 4.2: A Pressure Profile is Obtained by Drawing a Probe Down from the Rectum through the Anal Canal and Taking Recordings at 1 cm intervals. The physiological length of the anal canal is 3-3.5 cm and the pressure developed within it is largely due to the tonic activity of the internal sphincter.

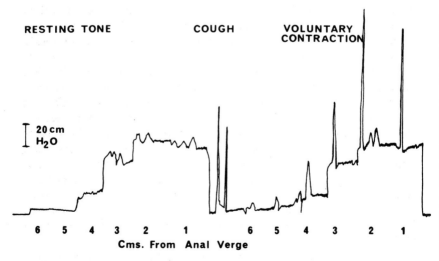

RESTING TONE   COUGH   VOLUNTARY CONTRACTION

20 cm H₂O

6   5   4   3   2   1   6   5   4   3   2   1
Cms. From Anal Verge

The maximal pressure is found half-way along the internal sphincter and is in the region of 60-80 cm of water. Distention of the rectum with, for instance, an air-filled balloon produces transient relaxation of the internal sphincter.[4-7] This reflex relaxation has been observed in patients with a cauda equina lesion, lesions of the sacral roots and after transection of the spinal cord.[8, 9] Serial distention of the rectum with small volumes produces a gradual increase in rectal pressure.[10] As the volume increases so does the occurrence of rectal contraction waves, whose frequency (nine cycles per minute) and amplitude (15 cm of water) remain more or less constant. Transient relaxation of the internal sphincter recurs after each increment is added (Figure 4.3). With each increment the base line pressure falls and after about 150-200 ml the internal sphincter completely relaxes, the balloon descends into the anal canal and only minimal straining is required to expel it. In patients with Hirschsprung's disease the reflex is absent and the internal sphincter fails to relax at all (Figure 4.4).[11] In this condition the intrinsic neural plexus of the rectum is abnormal, which suggests that the receptor site is in the viscus itself.

The Somatic Component

The skeletal muscles of the pelvic floor have a dual role; they combat the force of intra-abdominal pressure, thus preventing a pelvic hernia, and the external sphincter group (which includes the pubo-rectalis muscle) plays the most important part in the maintenance of continence. Muscles which are actuated only by voluntary means would be useless for the task of maintaining continence or of combatting gravitational forces, as the person's attention would need to be constantly drawn to them. An automatic mechanism is essential. If an electromyographic needle is inserted into most skeletal muscle no electrical activity at all is found at rest; it only develops as a result of voluntary or synergistic activity (Figure 4.5). The pelvic floor is quite different; the muscles are constantly contracting at rest and even during sleep.[12] But this is not all as, by means of automatic reflex action, the muscles will either additionally contract or relax according to appropriate circumstances.[6] Thus, when intra-abdominal pressure rises as a result of coughing,[13, 14] walking, lifting, etc., there is rapid reinforcement of the tonic activity of the pelvic floor muscles to resist this pressure (Figure 4.6). Voluntary contraction can be sustained for about 60 seconds but not much longer, after which activity fades[13] (see Chapter 1, p. 19).

Distention of the rectum by a balloon first increases the activity of the muscles. This again will protect against involuntary evacuation. When inflated to a greater size, reflex relaxation of the entire sphincter mass occurs.[8] This rarely occurs in normal circumstances. It is seen, however when there is impaction of faeces, such as occurs in patients

Figure 4.3: Anal Pressures are Recorded as a Balloon is Distended within the Rectal Ampulla. With each increment in the balloon, the tone of the internal sphincter decreases.

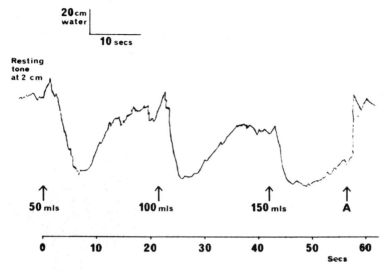

Figure 4.4: The Same Investigation is Performed as in Figure 4.3 but in This Case the Patient has Hirschsprung's Disease. There is no relaxation in the internal sphincter.

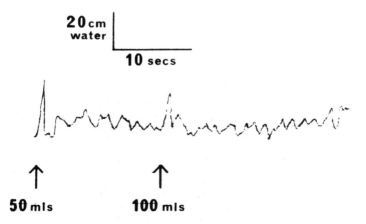

Figure 4.5: The Lower Recording is an Electromyographic Recording from the Extensor Muscles of the Forearm. At rest there is no activity at all. However, when the muscles are tensed, then activity commences, only to cease when the effort is finished. The upper recording shows an electromyogram of the external sphincters and it will be seen that activity is continuous and not dependent upon any voluntary effort. The latter can be superimposed but can only be sustained for about one minute.

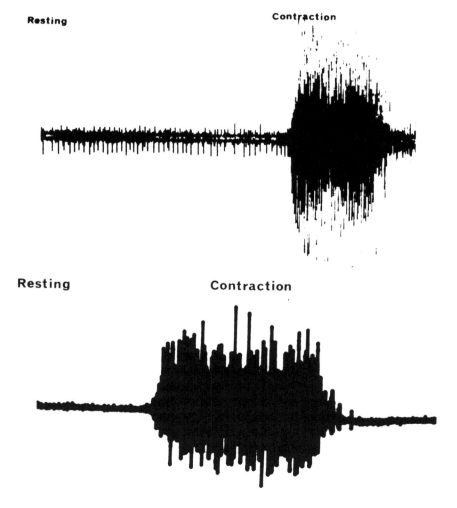

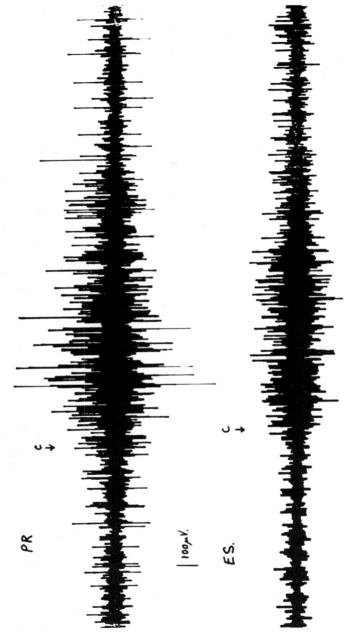

Figure 4.6: The Increased Electromyographic Activity in the Pelvic Floor during Coughing (C).

Key: PR, pubo-rectalis; ES, subcutaneous external sphincter

with idiopathic megacolon, in elderly people and in certain post-operative states. Here the rectum is grossly overloaded and the external sphincters are totally patulous. The main complaint of such a patient will be incontinence; he has no control at all. Liquid stool passing around the impacted mass leaks out without let or hindrance. This interesting physiological state is also a very practical one, demanding vigilance on the part of the doctor looking after the elderly patient. Fortunately, it is readily corrected.

Normal defaecation straining also inhibits the activity of the pelvic floor reflex[6, 14] and allows a stool to be passed without difficulty (Figure 4.7). However, if a person indulges in excessive defaecation straining over years, the pelvic floor is forced downwards at the same time as the muscles are relaxed and not counteracting this force. They are therefore passively stretched. Though recovery is almost certainly complete after a temporary episode of this nature, if the habit persists for years, the pelvic floor will be gradually forced lower and the muscles become stretched.[15] Not only may the muscles lengthen and become less efficient because of this, but the nerves supplying them are also stretched,[16, 17] in particular the branches supplying the external sphincter. This will be referred to later.

Figure 4.7: Attempt at Defaecation Causes Inhibition of the Skeletal Muscles of the Pelvic Floor. At the end of the effort there is a temporary burst of increased activity.

RESTING   STRAIN   REBOUND

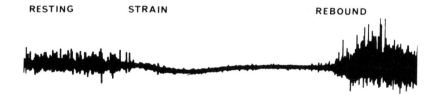

A mechanical valve effect is maintained by the tonic contraction of the external sphincters and pubo-rectalis muscles. The lower rectum makes a double right angle just before and on entering the upper anal canal (Figure 4.8). As a result, the upper part of the canal is closed by the anterior wall of the lower rectum, which impinges upon it. Any increase in abdominal pressure will automatically force that part of the lower rectal wall even more firmly upon the closed upper anal canal and will block it provided the anal sphincters remain active. In this way a flap valve is formed between a zone of high and low pressure.[1] Thus, any increase in abdominal pressure due to coughing, walking, etc., will automatically seal the upper anal canal and prevent faecal stress incontinence occurring. The angulation between the anal canal and lower rectum is maintained by the pubo-rectalis muscle.

Figure 4.8: The Anatomical Arrangement at the Ano-rectal Junction Results in the Formation of a Flap Valve. The anterior wall of the lower rectum impinges upon the closed anal canal and any increase in abdominal pressure seals the valve more securely.

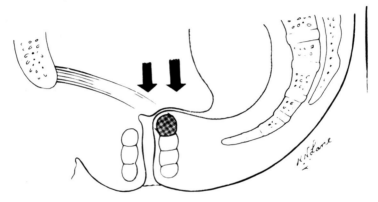

Sensation

Assessment of any sensation, whether qualitative or quantative, is always difficult. However, there is no doubt that in the normal person rectal distention produces a sensation of fullness in the perineum associated with a feeling of impending evacuation.[10] Distention above the ampulla produces only intestinal abdominal colic. It was originally thought that receptors responsible for 'rectal' sensation were present in the rectal wall. Recently, however, it has been shown that the sensory mechanism remains intact even after total excision of the rectum with anastomosis of the colon to the upper anal canal.[18] It is therefore apparent that the rectum itself is not the site of sensory information. The rectal ampulla lies in a cradle formed by the levator-ani muscles and it is probable that changes in volume stimulate stretch receptors in these muscles.

There are many causes of faecal incontinence. Table 4.1 lists the commoner ones, which will now be discussed in more detail.

Table 4.1: Causes of Faecal Incontinence

A. Severe diarrhoea:
  1. Ulcerative colitis
  2. Crohn's disease
  3. Diverticulitis
  4. Villous papilloma of the rectum
  5. Carcinoma of the rectum

B. Physiological disturbance:
  Impaction of faeces

C. Neurological disease:
  1. Cauda equina syndrome
  2. Other central nervous system disorders, including disseminated sclerosis
  3. Neuropathic change in the nerves supplying the pelvic floor muscles

D. Deficiency of the muscle ring:
  1. Ano-rectal agenesis
  2. Traumatic section

Severe Diarrhoea

Sudden, explosive diarrhoea may well cause an episode of incontinence even in a normal person. If, in addition, the subject has any pelvic floor defect, whether this be due to injury, neurological disease or the process of ageing, then they will be much more susceptible to such relatively minor events. A frequent cause of this state of affairs is inflammatory disease of the bowel, particularly diverticulitis. A villous papilloma secreting considerable quantities of mucus can have the same effect, as indeed can a carcinoma. These possibilities must always be borne in mind when dealing with a patient who is partially or totally incontinent. Provided that no organic disease is present, a patient can often be rendered symtpom-free by the simple process of inducing a more solid stool. This can be done by dietary means or by the use of one of the well-known drugs having a delaying action on the intestine. It is important to avoid the converse situation as the straining efforts required to evacuate a constipated stool will weaken the pelvic floor muscles even more.

Physiological Disturbance Accompanying Chronic Rectal Distention

Impaction of faeces is seen in the young patient with idiopathic megacolon, after surgery as well as in elderly people. Psychological factors are often implicated in the young but this is seldom the case and the child will almost always respond to corrective physical measures. The colon and rectum lack the necessary *vis a tergo* to propel faecal contents. A patient may be normal for years but a temporary enforced bed-rest due to illness may set a vicious cycle into action. The rectum becomes overloaded and it is impossible for such a mass to be evacuated normally. As we have seen, the sphincters lose their tone due to reflex inhibition. The child is incontinent, constantly soiling his clothing. This can go on for many years before treatment is instituted. First the impacted mass must be removed and this generally requires a general anaesthetic. The distended colon is atonic and will require stimulation to restore its activity. Disposable enemas are therefore given daily for a week to ten days. Thereafter one or more glycerine suppositories are given each day after breakfast to induce rectal contraction. This regime may be required for several months. In the post-operative patient, evacuation followed by suppositories for a few days will usually suffice.

In older people the problem is more complex, as the sphincter activity may be partially lost before impaction occurs. Such people will often keep the stool hard to maintain normal continence. It is easy then for them to be tripped over into impaction. Incontinence is an even more marked feature than with the other groups. When examined the anal canal may be gaping and patulous; once evacuated, however, sphincter tone returns. Patients may need a suppository routine almost indefinitely to prevent recurrence.

Neurological Disease

As reflex control of the pelvic floor is centred in the region of the cauda equina, lesions above this level, though capable of removing the conscious element, seldom cause grave impairment of function. Even in the case of a complete transection of the cord, reflex emptying of the rectum occurs once the stage of spinal shock has passed. Such patients learn how to induce reflex rectal contraction, usually by stimulating the lower anal canal.

Without doubt, the most difficult neurological situation to manage is the cauda equina syndrome. If the lesion is complete, there is no muscle activity in the pelvic floor at all, nor is there sensation.[19] These patients are totally incontinent. If they try to alleviate the situation by inducing a hard dehydrated stool, then they frequently become impacted. It is therefore usually necessary for them to keep the stool firm but to induce defaecation with the aid of glycerine suppositories or even disposable enemata.

Another category of neurologically-caused incontinence used to be given the title of 'idiopathic'. The most obvious feature of this condition is that the sphincter muscles are lax and patulous on clinical examination. Careful assessment reveals absence of an anal reflex, and no activity in the external sphincter itself. The pubo-rectalis muscle usually contracts on voluntary effort and the activity in the levator muscles may be within normal limits. There is, however, loss of tone in the pubo-rectalis muscle with the result that the normal ano-rectal angulation is lost and the efficiency of the flap valve mechanism is impaired.[1]

Physiological testing of the sphincters usually shows that no power at all is developed at rest either by the internal or external sphincter muscles.[20] The pressures developed on voluntary contraction vary greatly but are usually considerably less than normal.[3, 20] Routine electromyography is not grossly abnormal. Biopsy of the various muscles constituting the pelvic floor has revealed changes characteristic of degeneration in the nerves supplying the muscles.[16, 17] These changes are very similar to those found in the carpal tunnel syndrome at the wrist and indicate a local neuropathy. This is believed to be due to stretching of the nerves supplying the pelvic floor either by straining efforts over many years or in some cases the result of a difficult labour. A similar change is seen in association with rectal prolapse and here too the likely cause is pelvic floor descent resulting in lengthening and secondary degeneration of nerves supplying the sphincter muscles. It is this neuropathic change which can be detected by single fibre electromyography.[21]

The muscle degeneration in these patients is most severe in the external sphincter with increasing function present as one ascends through the pubo-rectalis muscle to the levator-ani group. The tone in the pubo-rectalis is grossly deficient so that the ano-rectal angulation is impaired.[15] Nevertheless, some activity in this muscle remains and it can be used to restore almost normal function in these patients. Should the patient have a large rectal prolapse, then this is first dealt with by means of a rectopexy. After this operation about one-third of patients will still be incontinent and they will need an operative repair of their pelvic floor exactly in the same way as those patients previously categorised as having idiopathic incontinence.

Any operation designed to relieve this condition must take into account the fact that the muscles are manifestly weakened and must aim at making the residual function maximally effective. An essential part of any procedure must be the reconstruction of the ano-rectal angulation, with restoration of the flap valve mechanism.[1] This objective can be obtained by reconstructing the pelvic floor muscles from behind the rectum and anal canal. The principle of the operative technique is to lift the visceral component of the anal canal forwards, off the inner surface of the anal sphincters, the pubo-rectalis and levator-ani muscles, and to place sutures from side to side across these muscles to shorten their effective length of action. At the same time the repair will restore the ano-rectal angle by approximating the two limbs of the pubo-coccygeus and pubo-rectalis muscles. The technique may be difficult and it would be inappropriate to discuss it in detail.[22] However, the mode of access to carry out this procedure is one of great anatomical interest. Advantage is taken of the previously-mentioned intersphincteric plane of embryological fusion between the viscus and the somatic muscles surrounding it. Through an incision performed behind the anal canal, the space between the internal and external sphincters is identified (Figure 4.9).

Figure 4.9: In the Operation of Post-Anal Repair of the Pelvic Floor Muscles and Anal Sphincters the First Step is to Dissect in the Intersphincteric Plane between the Visceral and Somatic Structures

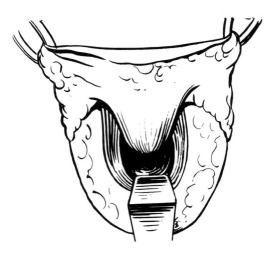

Figure 4.10: The Pelvis has been Entered by Dividing Waldeyer's Fascia. The ileo-coccygeus and pubo-coccygeus muscles are exposed.

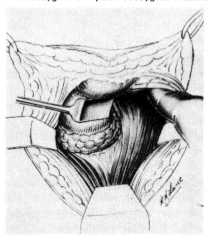

Figure 4.11 : Sutures are placed across the Pelvis between the Limbs of the Levator Muscles

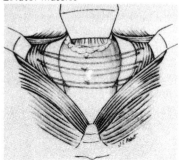

Figure 4.12: The Two Limbs of the Pubo-coccygeus and Pubo-rectalis Muscles are Approximated as Seen in this Diagram

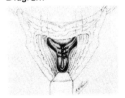

This plane is then opened up by a careful dissection and the internal sphincter is lifted off the skeletal muscles posteriorly and laterally. In succession the external sphincter is identified, the pubo-rectalis and (after division of Waldeyer's fascia) the pubo-coccygeus and ileo-coccygeus muscles (Figure 4.10). The plane is a bloodless one and no nerves cross it. Sutures are layed across from one limb of each exposed muscle to the other, starting with the ileo-coccygeus. About four layers of sutures are placed in descending order until the external sphincter is reached (Figure 4.11). By far the most important layers are in the pubo-coccygeus and pubo-rectalis muscles (Figure 4.12).

Post-operatively these patients either have a temporary colostomy to prevent disruption of the repair or are given artificially-induced diarrhoea for about ten to twelve days. Once this period has passed, the repair is sound. The need for careful management of these patients never ceases. If they return to their previous straining habits, the muscles will gradually lengthen again and they will revert to a similar state as they were in pre-operatively. It is therefore essential that evacuation is induced each day with the aid of an evacuant suppository (such as glycerine). They are also encouraged to perform sphincter exercises routinely, though this is probably only effective in the long term. It is very important to explain to the patient precisely the nature of the original condition and the measures required to prevent its recurrence.

Over 175 patients have been treated with this technique since 1959. Only ten per cent are men and the commonest age at operation is between 50 and 70 years. The condition, however, is not as uncommon in younger age groups as is usually supposed; the reason is that such people conceal their symptoms (as previously described). The operation gives satisfactory results in about 85 per cent of patients, which is not an unreasonable result bearing in mind the degree of atrophy which exists in the muscles. Success is defined as the ability of the patient to control a solid stool and to live a normal life without the need for padding, etc. Minor difficulties in coping with flatus and diarrhoea are not taken as indications of failure.

Deficiency of the Muscle Ring

Ano-rectal Agenesis

This is a subject requiring specialised experience and skill. A general principle is that only pelvic floor muscle can be used in any restorative operation, as only this has the tonic activity previously described. Despite apparent difficulties, it is important to realise that children who are afflicted can often be helped and, if not restored to complete normality, at least to a state of affairs which is manageable.

Traumatic Section

Trauma causing section of the muscle ring with retraction of muscle ending up to 180° is found associated with childbirth, surgery for anal fistula and automobile accidents. The female pelvic floor is particularly susceptible to muscle damage, incontinence following a degree of damage which would not cause symptoms in the male. The injury of childbirth is dealt with reasonably successfully by immediate reconstruction of the anterior perineum. A proportion fail, however, and these require formal reconstruction as a secondary procedure. Sphincter injury may also be caused by automobile and other forms of trauma, including operative treatment for anal fistula. In the past pessimism has been expressed regarding the results of reconstructional surgery in such cases, particularly when the defect was in the lateral or posterior site. However, provided there has been no neurological damage to the muscles, a satisfactory functional repair can almost always be achieved, no matter how bizarre the injury. It is essential to mobilise the ends of the divided muscle, freeing it from scar tissue binding it down to the fascia in the ischio-rectal fossa. To achieve a satisfactory result, overlap of the muscle ends without tension is essential and the repair is usually protected by a temporary colostomy[23] (Figure 4.13).

Our knowledge of the physiology and pathophysiology of the pelvic floor has greatly increased over the last 20 years. Most of the causes of incontinence can now be classified and their scientific basis is known. By one method or another most of them can be helped to overcome this very severe social disability. Equally important is the need for steps to be taken to prevent the causes of incontinence which set in with advancing age. The dietary habits of Western civilisation over the last hundred years have resulted in a high proportion of our people having to expel a hard stool with considerable difficulty. The straining efforts undoubtedly result in the neuropathic changes which we have described. It would be far better to prevent such changes occurring than to treat them once fully developed. It is therefore essential to educate the population to new dietary habits so that a more normal pattern of defaecation occurs spontaneously. The influence of childbirth on this condition is at present unknown, though strongly suspected in certain cases. Correction of difficulties during labour may well be another important factor we should be considering.

Figure 4.13: In Order to Achieve a Satisfactory Reconstruction Following Accidental Division of the Anal Sphincters, Extensive Dissection is Necessary and an Overlapping Repair is Performed

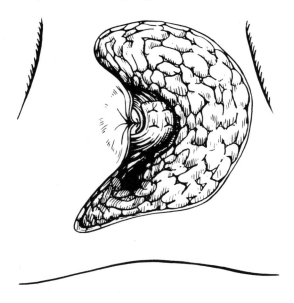

Notes

1. Parks, A.G. (1975), 'Anorectal Incontinence', *Proc. R. Soc. Med., 68,* 681.

2. Duthie, H.L. and Gairns, F.W. (1960), 'Sensory Nerve Endings and Sensation in the Anal Region of Man', *Br. J. Surg., 47,* 585-95.

3. Read, N.W., Harford, W.V., Schmulen, A.C., Read, M.G., Santa Ana, C. and Fordran, J.S. (1979), 'A Clinical Study of Patients with Faecal Incontinence and Diarrhoea', *Gastroenterology, 76,* 747-56.

4. Denny-Brown, D. and Robertson, E.G. (1935), 'An Investigation of the Nervous Control of Defaecation', *Brain, 58,* 256-310.

5. Gaston, E.A. (1948), 'The Physiology of Faecal Continence', *Surg. Gynec. Obstet., 87,* 280-90.

6. Parks, A.G., Porter, N.H. and Melzak, J. (1962), *Dis. Colon and Rectum, 5,* 407-14.

7. Schuster, M.M., Hendrix, T.R. and Mendeoff, A.I. (1963), 'The Internal Anal Sphincter Response: Manometric Studies on its Normal Physiology, Neural Pathways and Alteration in Bowel Disorders', *J. Clin. Invest., 42,* 196-207.

8. Melzak, J. and Porter, N.H. (1964), 'Studies of the Reflex Activity of

the External Sphincter Ani in Spinal Man', *Paraplegia, 1*, 277-96.
  9. Frenckner, B. (1975), 'Function of the Anal Sphincters in Spinal Man', *Gut, 16*, 638-44.
  10. Ihre, T. (1974), 'Studies on Anal Function in Continent and Incontinent Patients', *Scand. J. Gastroent., 9*, supp. 25.
  11. Aaronson, I. and Nixon, H.H. (1972), 'A Clinical Evaluation of Anorectal Pressure Studies in the Diagnosis of Hirschsprung's Disease', *Gut, 13*, 138-46.
  12. Floyd, W.F. and Walls, E.W. (1953), 'Electromyography of the Sphincter Ani Externus in Man', *J. Physiol., 122*, 599-609.
  13. Phillips, S.F. and Edwards, D.A.W. (1965), 'Some Aspects of Anal Continence and Defaecation', *Gut, 6*, 396-406.
  14. Kerrimans, R. (1969), *Morphological and Physiological Aspects of Anal Continence and Defaecation* (Editions Arscia, Brussels).
  15. Parks, A.G., Porter, N.H. and Hardcastle, J.D. (1966), 'Syndrome of the Descending Perineum', *Proc. R. Soc. Med., 59*, 477-82.
  16. Parks, A.G., Swash, M. and Urich, H. (1977), 'Sphincter Denervation in Ano-rectal Incontinence and Rectal Prolapse', *Gut, 18*, 656-65.
  17. Beersiek, F., Parks, A.G. and Swash, M. (1979), 'Pathogenesis of Ano-rectal Incontinence: A Histometric Study of the Anal Sphincter Musculature', *J. Neurol. Sci., 42*, 111-27.
  18. Lane, R.H.S. and Parks, A.G. (1977), 'Function of the Anal Sphincters Following Colo-anal Anastomosis', *Br. J. Surg., 64*, 596-99.
  19. Walton, J.N. (1977), *Brain's Diseases of the Nervous Sytem* (Oxford University Press, Oxford).
  20. Henry, M.M. and Parks, A.G. (1980), 'The Investigation of Anorectal Function', *Hospital Update* (January).
  21. Neill, M.E. and Swash, M. (1980), 'Increased Motor Unit Fibre Density in the External and Anal Sphincter Muscle in Ano-rectal Incontinence: A Single Fibre EMG Study', *J. Neurol. Neurosurg. Psychiat.*, in press.
  22. Parks, A.G. (1977), 'Post-anal Pelvic Floor Repair' in Rob, C., Smith, R. and Morgan, C.M. (eds.), *Operative Surgery*, 3rd edn (Butterworth, London).
  23. Parks, A.G. and McPartlin, J.F. (1971), 'Late Repair of Injuries of the Anal Sphincter', *Proc. R. Soc. Med., 64*, 1187-9.

5 INCONTINENCE IN GENERAL MEDICAL PATIENTS

G.S.C. Sowry

Urinary (and less frequently, faecal) incontinence is a major factor in the decision-making management activities of a general physician, if only because a high proportion of the cases under his care are elderly. This immediately brings the question of age into the discussion of the problem.

It is as well to remember that continence is an acquired, and not a congenital, habit. For a period of between one and three years at the beginning of their lives, human beings do not possess the ability to control when they will micturate; or if they do possess it, they are not motivated to put it into effect. These two attributes of continence — mechanical ability and motivation — are constantly to the forefront in any consideration of incontinence and in many cases physicians have to make an initial assessment as to which of these two factors is primarily at fault. The decision of this dilemma is not always easy, for in ill-health both may be involved. Correspondingly, in cases of 'organic' inability to control micturition the inability may be only partial and capable of being overcome by determined motivation (see Chapter 12).

The value of the individual (and thus to the survival of the species) of continence is obvious. Comfort, social custom, good hygiene (and therefore lessened risk of infections), the ability to keep warm by wearing clothes — all of these would be at risk if incontinence prevailed in the human race. Indeed, it requires no great leap from this thought to realise that the organised social structure of man's life (of varying degrees of sophistication) would never have come about if continence of both urine and faeces had not been acquired. (It is to be noted, at this point, that man is not the only animal capable of continence — domestic pets are not assured of domestic survival if regularly or frequently incontinent. In other highly developed mammals, continence presumably confers no advantage and has perhaps not been acquired — it is to be doubted whether the whale or the porpoise has evolved this skill!)

From this general consideration of the value of continence to the race or to the individual, the converse can be seen more clearly; namely the disadvantages of incontinence. Put in its most acute form, the future care of an elderly patient may be largely determined by his or her ability or inability to control micturition and defaecation. Inability will necessitate a greater degree of nursing and social care than can be provided in most private or 'welfare' homes, and will often necessitate a hospital or equivalent environment for the patient (see Chapter 13). Incontinence has been classified and the mechanisms necessary for continence have been described in Chapters 1, 2, 3 and 4. The most common causes of incontinence in general medical patients involve one or more of the following primary factors:

(1) impairment or loss of consciousness;
(2) impairment of volition;
(3) malfunction or interruption of controlling neurological pathways;
(4) mechanical derangement of bladder or bowel sphincters.

In addition there are a number of conditioning or secondary factors:

(5) hyperactivity of voiding reflexes;
(6) increased volume (of urine or faeces) to be voided.

A few examples of these mechanisms will now be described.

The State of Consciousness

Severe strokes or head injuries generally result in incontinence (or perhaps in retention with overflow which in effect is incontinence). The relative 'survival' benefit of this as compared with urinary or faecal obstruction is obvious.

Volition

The wish to be dry and clean can lapse or disappear in confusional states, depression, dementia and a great many other conditions. It is commonly diminished in sickness and old age, so that unpleasant or distressing factors in another field may combine with the diminished desire for continence to produce the reverse. Quite minor adverse conditioning factors which can with thought be avoided or corrected may result in incontinence. For example an unpleasantly low temperature in the lavatory or (paradoxically) a wet or slippery floor may make all the difference between continence and incontinence in an elderly or mildly-confused patient. Similar a lavatory that has to be approached by stairs or is at a distance may result in incontinence because the patient dislikes the discomfort of reaching the lavatory more than he or she dislikes being wet or dirty.

Consideration should always be given to ways by which a faltering volition can be reinforced. In general such methods fall into the categories of rewards or punishments (incentives or disincentives). The most simple forms, but often the most effective, are praise on the one hand and an expression of disapproval on the other. Often the reward or the punishment is a built-in part of the situation. The patient who wishes to get back to his or her home but who cannot do so as long as incontinence persists is a clear example, so long as the situation has been truthfully explained. A hundred years ago it was not uncommon for boys (and perhaps less commonly girls) to be 'encouraged' to develop continence by means of the whip. The natural development of continence in children perhaps persuaded those who used it of the effectiveness of their treatment. Who is to deny that occasionally, in lazy children, the treatment was effective?

No one in their senses would now advocate disincentives which involve pain or cruelty. But what can be said of allowing the patient, whom one believes to be capable of continence given more volition, to 'stew in his own juice' for a bit? The converse can be even more effective, namely arranging for the patient to wear a favourite suit or dress. This can be a powerful incentive (see Chapter 12).

Any discussion of the role of volition in this field would be incomplete without a consideration of drugs. Indeed drugs could equally have been included in the previous section on consciousness. Many sedatives, hypnotics and tranquillisers are to blame for persistent or resurgent incontinence. Alcohol is a double offender, for not only may it impair consciousness and volition but also it will increase the 'voidable' load and stimulus. This is not to deny the use of such agents in appropriate cases, but it is necessary to bear in mind the possibility of incontinence being attributable to it.

The problem arises, therefore, as to what we should prescribe for a patient who complains of sleeplessness but who is at risk of becoming incontinent if night sedatives or hypnotics are employed. The answer is, of course, that the minimal quantity of the mildest agent should be used. For those who are used to it, and who enjoy it, a whisky 'night cap' is as good a remedy as any. Where there is an element of anxiety, a tranquilliser such as diazepam may help; others may prefer nitrazepam, but its tendency to provoke alarming dreams may be a disadvantage. Whatever is used, two important rules should be observed. First, the patient should micturate immediately before going to sleep and secondly, the degree of sedation should not be so great as to prevent the patient from micturating in a 'controlled' manner if he or she wakes in the night with the desire to do so.

Malfunction of Neurological Control

The normal mechanisms by which the bladder and the rectum are emptied of their stored contents have been discussed elsewhere (Chapters 1 and 4). Malfunction of these mechanisms can result either in augmentation of the voiding stimulus or in interference with the stimulus or with the response to it.

Pathological augmentation of the stimulus occurs in a number of conditions. Epilepsy of the *grand mal* variety characteristically results in urinary and, occasionally, in faecal, incontinence, which is due to the abnormal and widespread discharge of neurological stimuli. A similar, but usually less marked, event may occur in sudden vagal stimulation as with a simple vaso-vagal attack or in a more sinister event such as myocardial infarction or pulmonary embolus.

Marked emotional stimulation can result in incontinence. 'God speed', said the lady as she broke the champagne bottle over the bows of the ship which she was launching. 'So have I, mummy' said her small son, standing beside her, 'I was so excited.'

Neurological lesions which interefere with or suppress the reflexes include:

Cerebral lesions. It is comparatively rare for strokes or other cerebral lesions to cause incontinence unless the lesion has also caused impairment of consciousness and/or volition. The patient whose stroke results solely in a motor hemiparesis usually remains continent.

Cord Lesions. These, if complete (paraplegia) most commonly result in retention of urine with overflow. It is generally necessary to catheterise such patients; the risk of urinary tract infection is less from catheterisation (hygienically carried out) than from permanent retention. The risk of pressure sores is, of course, greatly increased by incontinence.

Partial or slowly progressive cord lesions, as in multiple sclerosis, generally result in urgency of micturition or defaecation, with increased frequency of either and the risk of incontinence if suitable facilities are not readily available.

Peripheral Nerve Lesions. These, of necessity, must involve the autonomic system. Diabetic autonomic neuropathy can cause frequency of micturition, sometimes with incontinence, and of defaecation where, inexplicably as yet, there is often also diarrhoea. Classically this is often worse at night and may result in faecal incontinence.

Occasionally distressing faecal incontinence can result from a failure of rectal sensation. To those who have not thought of it, it may come as a surprise when they consider the remarkably accurate sensory perception that normally prevails as to whether the rectal contents are gaseous, solid or liquid. Failure in this sensory discrimination, be it transient (e.g. from alcohol or drugs) or permanent (from neurological damage to the sensory pathways) may lead to faecal incontinence (see Chapter 4).

Mechanical Factors

The tone, anatomy and function of the sphincter mechanisms (both urinary and faecal) and the physical condition of related structures need to be considered. These topics are discussed elsewhere in this book, but it is necessary to mention them in this chapter dealing with incontinence as seen by a general physician, if only because these factors are so frequently involved in incontinence, wherever it occurs.

The most frequent of these types of urinary incontinence is that due to pelvic floor laxity in the female. Treatment by surgical correction, by mechanical supports for the pelvic floor, by special pelvic floor exercises, and by stimulatory excitation of the affected muscles are the most effective lines of treatment (see Chapters 3 and 10).

Prostatic hypertrophy, benign or malignant, causes its earliest symptoms by enhancing the urinary voiding reflex. As a result, frequency and urgency of micturition are presenting features. A diminution of urinary stream and 'dribbling' at the end of micturition follow, and lead in due course to retention of urine with overflow incontinence (see Chapters 1 and 2).

Pressure upon the bladder from pelvic masses (e.g. fibroids, or faecal distention of the rectum) may lead to urinary incontinence as may physical lesions of the bladder itself (see Chapters 3 and 4). Faecal incontinence can result from mechanical defects in the anal sphincter in a similar way , although it is far less common (see Chapter 4).

Local Enhancement of Voiding Reflexes

So far this chapter has dealt with basic defects which directly cause incontinence. It is necessary now to consider some more indirect mechanisms.

Increasing pressure on the sole of a normal foot will eventually lead to a reflex withdrawal of the foot from the stimulus: if the foot is for any reason inflamed, a lesser pressure will evoke the response. The same is true of the bladder and of the rectum. Local inflammation (cystitis or proctitis) will enhance the voiding reflex, and if the enhancement is sufficient, or the patient's volition weak, incontinence may well result.

It follows that urinary tract infections, so common in patients confined to bed, can lead to incontinence. The story is so common as to be almost expected in elderly patients. The mechanisms involved include many of those that have already been mentioned in this chapter.

Consider the case of an elderly woman admitted with an acute respiratory infection. This will lead to drowsiness (impaired volition). She will be nursed in bed and will develop general and local muscle weakness (loss of sphincter tone). She will tend to become constipated with consequent mechanical pressure on the bladder. Urinary infection will lead to cystitis (enhanced voiding reflex).

Forty years ago a well-known *viva* question to medical students was 'What action would you take if an elderly patient with pneumonia becomes incontinent?' The correct answer was: 'Send for the relatives.' Antibiotics have rendered this answer less cogent today. But incontinence is still a common indication that things are not going well. With forethought and correct attention to the factors involved, this type of incontinence and the adverse prognosis it heralds should be preventable in many cases. Where it does occur, correction of the various factors (including the urinary infection) will bring benefit.

This section would not be complete without mentioning that lesions of the bladder or rectum other than inflammation can cause the same effects, for example trauma or neoplastic infiltration.

Increased Volume of Urine or Faeces

Throughout this chapter, the interplay of the various factors determining continence or incontinence has been stressed. Into this complicated series of equations must now be introduced the bulk or volume to be voided; clearly any increase in this will tend to tip the scales towards incontinence, all other things being equal.

To consider urinary incontinence first, increased urine volume can result from a number of general medical conditions, which will now be discussed.

Treatment with Diuretics

The response of a patient to diuretics will depend upon a number of factors which include the excess, and therefore voidable, volume of extracellular fluid and the responsiveness of the kidneys to the diuretic. As an example, a relatively youthful patient with previously untreated congestive cardiac failure may well have profuse diuresis in response to a single dose of a mild diuretic, e.g. thiazide. If the patient is not so young and has a number of other factors tending to promote incontinence, this diuresis may well cause it. For this reason and because of the inconvenience of polynocturia (with or without incontinence) doctors are rightly advised where possible to avoid regimes of treatment which will lead to nocturia. But, if faced with a patient who, without treatment, will be kept awake by dyspnoea, the choice must surely be to treat with diuretics (which, of course, include any drug which relieves cardiac failure) whether or not this results in sleep disturbed by polyuria or in incontinence.

Disease-induced Nocturia

There are a number of disease processes which can lead spontaneously to nocturnal polyuria (and hence, in the conditionally predisposed to incontinence). One of the commonest is cardiac failure itself. The day of physical exertion is followed by the night of rest; increased demand upon the heart is followed by diminished demand, fluid retention by diuresis and oliguria (unnoticed by the patient) by polyuria. The elderly patient in this situation may well be troubled by 'restless' nights and, if the true cause is not spotted, may be prescribed more sedatives or more hypnotics. It is easy for incontinence to occur in these circumstances. The correct treatment is, of course, the use of a diuretic in the morning, so that the diurnal fluid retention and hence the nocturnal polyuria do not occur.

Other Causes of Polyuria

There are many causes of polyuria; examples are diabetes mellitus, diabetes insipidus (rare), chronic renal failure and polydipsia, which may be caused by obsessional neurosis. Diabetes mellitus is probably the commonest and in those predisposed to incontinence by age or other of the factors discussed may well cause incontinence. The clue to the correct diagnosis in such cases may well lie in the history of thirst, weight-loss, vulvitis, etc. But such clues may be absent. However, as the general examination of any patient should invariably include examination of the urine, this cause of incontinence should not escape detection by the conscientious doctor.

Chronic renal disease, including that induced by hypercalcaemia, may well be missed even if routine urine testing is carried out, but should generally be detected by a careful history and examination, and be confirmed by a simple biochemical investigation.

Obsessional polydipsia generally affects the young or middle-aged, and as a result, incontinence of urine must be a rare manifestation. Occasionally, however, the polydipsia is relatively mild and more the result of habit than of obsession. The appropriate treatment, where it is causing incontinence, is simply to discourage the habit.

Faecal incontinence is seldom due to increased stool bulk. However, diarrhoea is a common cause as is well known. An important variant is 'spurious diarrhoea' due to faecal impaction in the rectum. This gives rise to proctitis with large quantities of mucus being formed and frequently causes faecal incontinence (see Chapter 4, p. 86). Unless the true cause is detected, anti-diarrhoeal remedies, such as codeine or kaolin, may be given, whereupon the constipation is increased and the spurious diarrhoea and incontinence are increased. The diagnosis is made by rectal examination; the treatment is by enema, or whatever else is needed to relieve the impaction.

Other causes of diarrhoea which may result in faecal incontinence include infective enteritis or colitis, malabsorption syndromes, neoplasms of the large bowel, pancreatitis or pancreatic neoplasms. Rarely patients inflict the problem on themselves by addiction to purgatives, an addiction which they will usually attempt to conceal.

Conclusion

In this brief review of the problem of urinary and faecal incontinence as seen by a general physician, an attempt has been made to encourage a methodical approach to the question of causation.

Age, with its increasing liability to confusion and lessened volition, is by far the biggest factor. Mechanical malfunction of the sphincter mechanisms, especially of the bladder, is probably the second most important cause. The conditioning factors of cystitis or, less commonly, proctitis play a part as do polyuria and diarrhoea (true or spurious).

If the patient and his or her relatives are to be spared the tribulations which are attendant on incontinence, it behoves physicians to make an accurate assessment of its cause as a first step to its prevention or cure.

6A INCONTINENCE AND THE TEAM IN GERIATRIC MEDICINE

Monnica Stewart

There is no great mystique to the practice of geriatric medicine, contrary to the occasionally wishful modern medical thought. For there is no disease or pathology that only afflicts people who are aged over 65. All the illnesses that happen to people over that age can equally well occur in younger people, including even atherosclerosis which can start forming from the age of seven onwards.

Some years ago a famous British nurse in this field, Doreen Norton, remarked that a first-class sister of a geriatric medical ward could take over any other type of ward in any specialty and be equally excellent within two to four weeks (i.e. when she had learned the technological skills of the specialty). The practice of geriatric medicine requires not only the exercise of high professional skill and knowledge, backed by patience and willingness to contrive the integration of personal relationships with patients and their relatives and friends. It also needs the co-operation of a team of professional and voluntary workers to restore the patient to some form of personal independence. To quote Doreen Norton, 'Independence cannot be achieved independently' and a physician in geriatric medicine must catalyse the processes involved in the difficult path back to personal autonomy. As it has also been put: 'Enabling requires the capacity to be hopeful in circumstances that deny reason for hope.'[1]

The whole philosophy of this kind of medicine is summed up in a classic paper by Professor Bernard Isaacs in the *British Medical Journal*[2] which remains as pertinent now as when it was written:

Few diseases at any age are cured; most whisper to the patient of their continuing presence long after the ink is dry on the discharge letter. The treatment of the irremediable is both a worthy objective and accurate description of much of modern medicine.
It is amongst such disabled people that the doctor seeks opportunity for effective intervention.
Confusion and incontinence are symptoms of impaired function of the nervous system and bladder. The words give no information on cause or cure.

This brings us to the nub of difficulties experienced by people labelled geriatric and incontinent. Basically the difficulties are the same as those experienced by younger people who are incontinent, but with a difference — the difference being that the older person's problems are magnified disproportionately by the attitude of those around him and by his age and the limited choice of opportunities, facilities and consumer goods open to one who is no longer a wage-earner and one who is deemed to be without a meaningful future. Ceaselessly we proclaim that old people are no different from younger people except that they are likely to have more leisure because they are mostly retired from active employment and for the same reason are likely to have less financial resources. Similarly, because they have lived longer amid the hostile and adverse conditions of modern industrial society, they are likely to have more physical disabilities. There are no other real differences, yet the myth is perpetuated that the elderly are a race apart and their problems different from those of the rest of society and that separate people, facilities, expertise, and so forth are needed to deal with them. There is always a hint too, that the elderly and disabled are lazy and have to be continually prodded into activity, otherwise they will sit about expecting to be waited on. A good illustration of this line of thought is enshrined in *Hansard* for 21 May 1971 when the Minister of Health, then Sir Keith Joseph, was having to reply to a parliamentary question, presumably using the material prepared for him by his expert medical advisors. The subject under discussion was the provision of accessible inside lavatories for disabled people.

We know, alas, that many disabled people live in homes where they are separated either by stairs or by having to go outside their houses to get to lavatories. I am told that, medically, it can be very important to leave a motive for the disabled person to move and that, therefore, we should not jump to the conclusion that the provision of a lavatory conveniently, as we all enjoy, is necessarily good for such a person; I am sure that we would all take the view, but it may be that the stimulus to move is necessary for some.

It is difficult in the context of a book like this to believe such a crass theory could ever have been propounded by any doctor, but one knows that thinking of that nature unfortunately abounds amongst workers in the medical professions. There is no doctor, nurse, therapist, social or auxiliary worker, who has not at some time heard some variant on this depersonalising theme.

Yet fundamentally the most superb diagnosis and prescription of treatment and the use of sophisticated technology are only of proper value when accompanied by explanation and reassurance. There also needs to be the conviction on the recipient's part that all that can be done to minimise personal discomfort, has been done. An interesting aside on this is evidenced by the high level of dissatisfaction expressed by astronauts at the arrangements made for urine and faecal excretion and its disposal in spacecraft life. It is to be hoped that the scientific research being accomplished by NASA may have some spin-off for some of the more routine problems associated with the mechanical difficulties experienced by heavily-handicapped people, in dealing independently with their own excretory requirements.

As has been stated time and time again throughout this book, incontinence is an emotive topic and impatience, intolerance and distaste for it is the common reaction. Yet ingestion and excretion are the most fundamental and important of all human activities and perhaps are other reasons for the somewhat ironic description that one occasionally hears, of physicians in geriatric medicine being the 'guardians of the orifices'! Therefore any professional helper involved with the management of patients with atypical patterns must be prepared to undertake personal involvement and take time to listen. A ready ear at the right moment can save hours of frustration and mutual dissatisfaction between patient and would-be helper.

Once the mental leap has been achieved and incontinence has been accepted not as an inevitable accompaniment of ageing but as a symptom and also as a dire emergency for the patient, the steps to be taken are the same whoever is the first disciplinary team member on the scene. Comfort, support and remedial action for the patient and then assessment of the cause by the professional using Dorothy Mandelstam's check-list (see Appendix B) are needed. As so often in medical work the cause is frequently so ludicrously obvious, simple and easily remedied that one is ashamed to think how often it is not recognised. Instead the first emergency, inadequately managed, is allowed to drift into a routine mopping-up operation with consequent demoralisation of patient and supporting relatives or staff. Demoralisation of the patient is a personal disaster, but demoralisation of supporters has far wider implications and is given too little attention. Visit any women's general medical ward to see a specific patient and one can almost guarantee that a great many other patients passed *en route* will be asking for a bedpan or for help to be taken to the toilet. Staff look rueful and downcast when asked if the specific patient would be continent if there were enough pairs of hands to help her go to the toilet on a regular two-hourly basis. They are usually only too painfully aware that this simple remedy is beyond their capabilities within the current staffing provision (see Chapter 11, p. 171).

This frustrating by-product of staff shortage must prey on the mind of the conscientious nurse, and produce feelings of depression at the sheer inability to give the patients the basic routine care which they need to maintain dignity and independence. Facing situations like this daily can have only two possible outcomes: rebellion against the system or opting-out in sheer professional self-preservation. This opting-out can be literal by transfer to some other branch of nursing such as casualty, obstetrics, theatre or community work or else to another occupation altogether. This in itself produces problems for future staffing levels, but perhaps in some ways the worst form of opting-out is that of adopting the stereotyped attitude that incontinence is inevitable in an old person, and there is nothing one can do but put in a catheter or settle the patient on an incontinence pad.

It is towards prevention of this last form of opting-out that we must turn our efforts enthusiastically and many years of solid work will be required, for basic attitudes have to be changed by education, not only of professionals but also of the general public (see Chapter 7). Education has to be accompanied by boring repetition of the statement that *incontinence is not an inevitability of ageing or disability* and should never be met with passive acceptance. Maintenance of continence can be achieved by therapeutic positiveness and the recognition that the work required, particularly in an institutional setting, is a genuine team effort. Too long has it been considered to be only a nursing duty with which doctors and therapists should rarely meddle. As in the case of a completed stroke (so often used as a common denominator for so many variants of disability), there needs to be a very clear medical diagnosis in the first instance to ensure realistic endeavour and the wise words of Professor George Adams spring to mind:

> Persistent incontinence in the absence of local causes is a discouraging prognostic sign. It may be part of a picture of deteriorating intellect, or it may be associated with cerebral damage in the frontal area of the right (non-dominant) hemisphere. Recovery from incontinence related to lesions in the area seems to be unduly prolonged or, if associated with severe sensory deficit and anosognosia, to remain intractable.[3]

Provision of an accurate neurological assessment is therefore necessary on two counts — to prevent the labelling of a patient so afflicted as lazy or dirty and to protect enthusiastic staff from disappointment or from blaming the patient if intensive therapeutic efforts are not crowned with success.

Realism is as important in the maintenance of continence as it is in any other field of medical management, but it must be based on knowledge and understanding of the underlying processes rather than on mythology or traditional teaching aphorisms. Having made a diagnosis after careful history-taking, physical examination and investigation, and having evolved with appropriate team colleagues a suitable regime for each individual patient, the doctor's role of involvement does not then cease. He must remain interested, not only to support the staff, but also to ensure timely therapeutic intervention if drug treatment, or lack of it, is actually causing the loss of excretory control. The ill-judged use of potent diuretic or sedative, the lack of urinary antibiotic or even the lack of laxative, can all produce hazards for the patient (see Chapter 5, p. 100). For instance, few inexperienced prescribers are aware that iron can produce violent diarrhoea in some people and profound constipation in others, both of which could lead to faecal incontinence when linked to prolapsed rectum or immobility or some other disability in a particular patient.

Many a fine plan of management of incontinence has failed through lack of communication or discussion between all members of a supporting therapeutic team — between themselves or even with the patient. This can be so, whether it is at home or in an institutional setting. Working outwards from the involvement of the key figure of the patient, to relative, friend, neighbour or voluntary worker, one then needs to consider all the statutory workers. The nursing auxiliary, remedial helper, home-help and sometimes even the ward domestic, often need to be just as involved as the trained professional. How often, too, does communication fail between night and day helpers?

The role of the nurse in management is well chronicled and obvious; less obvious is the role of the therapist and the social workers. The physio/occupational therapist and nurse, between them will be concerned with mobility, muscle function and re-education, and with the ergonomics of bed, chair, commode, toilet space, heights of lavatory seats, positioning of grab handles and siting and type of toilet paper and holders. The occupational therapist, with the nurse, will be particularly concerned with the provision of appropriate, or where necessary, adapted clothing. The speech therapist has the specific role of establishing means of communication for the aphasic and dysarthric patient helping to ensure that he can obtain help when needed. The social worker (it was Joan Kenyon Rogers, a geriatric medical social worker, who first coined the phrase 'life is lived at the lavatory level'), is equally vital in the communication chain. It will often be the social worker who, with knowledge of the background culled from the patient, relatives, friends, home-helps or voluntary helpers, will also smooth the path for ultimate discharge from hospital, ensuring that the receiving environment will be right for maintenance of continence (see Chapter 13).

Words such as teamwork, integration, multidisciplinary co-operation, communication and co-operation glide smoothly from lip and pen, but the question remains, how do we bring all these things about on the hospital ward, in the residential home and at home where people live? How do we break through the sound barrier between word and actuality to the point where there really is a belief that the first incident of incontinence at any age (once toilet training has been accomplished) is a real emergency that calls for instant concern and alert questioning and, if needs be, investigation until the cause is elicited and the right remedial action taken?

There seems to be no easy path to the solution of the problems. The ripple phenomenon is endless. Architects have to rethink design of housing and public buildings in conjunction with ergonomists (see Chapter 7). Not only has there to be adequate lavatory provision at every level in buildings but it must be accessible, properly-designed and within easy distance of potential users. Public-transport designers have to reconsider provision of facilities as anyone will testify who has ever tried to assist a disabled or even an able-bodied but slightly-confused person in the toilet cubicle of an aeroplane, train or ship. Improvisation and adaptations are possible in many instances, but appropriate design in all new buildings is a far better policy. Meanwhile we must give more attention and allocate more resources to improving the equipment that is available and ensuring that it is instantly obtainable at the time of need. A survey by the Disabled Living Foundation and Age Concern (Greater London)[4] revealed that in Greater London many health districts had a waiting period of at least five days for the provision of commodes to patients at home. Very few had a full range of equipment that the community nurse could take to her patient at home once she had made her initial assessment of the situation. Concentration to date has been centred on distribution of incontinence pads and on laundry provision, although seldom is any thought given to the disposal of soiled incontinence items.

As in so many areas of health the emphasis now needs to be not on crisis intervention but on prophylaxis and on sensible measures to ensure that the present unpropitious climate, for elderly people and their gallant supporters, should alter. We all know that we have an ageing population, and that there is going to be a far higher percentage of people aged 85 and over than ever previously known. Judged by present standards and attitudes this could be a fearful prospect for this very vulnerable section of the population. If attitudes can be altered, if people's disabilities and requirements are assessed on an individual basis and not related to age groups or categories (see Chapter 12), if future planning and design are based on actual population needs, and resources are deployed from areas of high technology but limited patient utilisation, to areas of less exacting technology but high patient utilisation, then the economics of the future may be more hopeful.

Without such adjustment the future for the elderly incontinent patient can only be gloomy, for the custodian of yore, the omnipresent nurse, is becoming one of the scarcest resources and more and more institutions are closing their doors from lack of supporting staff. Battling with incontinence without the right support, equipment, or environment, is one of the major factors in professional and personal demoralisation of nursing staff. When this is allied to ageing patients and the traditional disparagement associated in industrial societies with all aspects of ageing it can only point to a crisis in the near future. Geriatric medicine has led the way in demonstrating that co-ordination of endeavour and multidisciplinary expertise can enable apparent miracles of return to personal independence to happen in the most unpromising conditions and situations. It now remains for the catalysts to continue in other specialties.

Notes

1. Taylor, J. (1979), *Social Work Today*, *11*, 20.
2. Isaacs, B. (1973), *Br. Med. J.*, *3*, 526-8.
3. Adams, G.F. (1974), *Cerebrovascular Disability and the Ageing Brain* (Churchill Livingstone, Edinburgh).
4. Age Concern (Greater London) (1979), *Improving Services for the Incontinent Adult* (Age Concern, London).

6B OLD PEOPLE AND DISORDERS OF CONTINENCE

Michael F. Green

Introduction

1. The elderly are not a homogenous group. Chronological and biological age are not the same, but the older old (i.e. over 75 or 80 years) are more likely as a group — but not as individuals — to suffer many acute and chronic problems, including disturbances of normal bladder and bowel function.

2. Incontinence is not an inevitable reflection of ageing, nor does it automatically imply dementia; senility is not a medical disease.

3. Expert, thorough history-taking and general and gynaecological examination and appropriate investigations are just as likely to be needed in older people with disturbed continence as in younger people — indeed, more so. This is because there are many causes of incontinence in old age, e.g. problems affecting bodily function and mobility, which can be aggravated by an unhelpful environment and drugs.

4. Old people tend to:

   (a) Accumulate multiple pathology, often interacting and summating with each other.

   (b) Acquire polypharmacy — both prescribed and bought over the counter (OTC) medicines, any of which can be harmful and may cause or aggravate incontinence.

   (c) Suffer from pathologies that have modified, atypical or completely non specific clinical pictures compared with the 'classical' medical presentation usually seen in younger people. Incontinence may be the final common pathway of many different underlying pathologies.

   (d) Manifest disease problems by functional disability affecting the elderly person's ability to lead a normal daily life and as a result of immobility and/or instability secondarily produce incontinence.

   (e) Develop, often insidiously a reduction in organ function and reserve capacity to deal with stress, e.g. affecting normal kidney, bladder or bowel function.

(f) Suffer from a reduction in normal homeostatic body balancing mechanisms. Normal balance and co-ordination, posture and gait, temperature control, blood pressure and blood sugar levels may not be normal at rest or when the body responds to normal activity. Again, the outward manifestation is likely to be functional disability such as an inability, falls or incontinence.

(g) Be more likely than many younger people to be hard up, to live in poor 'quality' housing with inadequate amenities, and to have no or few visiting supportive relatives and friends. Again, the consequence is a predisposition to and vulnerability to the effects of functional problems including disturbed incontinence.

Incontinence, particularly of urine, is one of the giants of geriatric medicine causing great distress, and often leading to demands for admission to 'institutional' care. It has been suggested that at least 20-25 per cent of people over 65 will become incontinent of urine frequently, even daily. This is obviously a major medical and nursing problem and causes great distress to many older people, and their carers. On the bright side, it can often be cured or controlled, should not lead to automatic admission to a home or hospital, and 75-80 per cent of old people are not incontinent. It cannot be reiterated too often to doctors, nurses and other health professionals as well as to old people and the general public that however embarrassing and unpleasant incontinence is when it develops in old people, it is not inevitably incurable, nor does it mark the onset of a mythical disease called senility. All too often it is assumed that the age of the person is the primary problem. In fact it is always the incontinence which is the problem and this will often have the same causes and, therefore, the same potential for medical or surgical cure as in younger people. However, it is true that the almost epidemic nature of incontinence in old age represents a problem in itself, and that there are many special aspects of the aetiology and management of incontinence in older people. A knowledge of paediatric and mesiatric incontinence problems cannot necessarily be automatically transposed to the management of older incontinent patients.

Not only is incontinence one of the giants of geriatric medicine but it may be caused by or complicate many of the other major functional problems such as immobility, instability, intellectual impairment, inadequate sensory input, or iatrogenic (doctor caused) disease. Repeatedly it must be emphasised that it is the individual's circumstances that determine the level of incontinence. Incontinence is not just due to stroke, dementia or diuretics as many people with these problems or taking other potentially incontinent-making drugs are not in fact incontinent.

The older the incontinence victim, the more likely it is that if the incontinence is not cured or 'cleanly' controlled, it is then likely to lead to the breakdown of the network of social support. This eventually means that the old person has to leave their home or residential home, their family and friends and be admitted to a nursing home or hospital often for good. The five dominant characteristics identified in elderly people admitted for prolonged geriatric care by Isaacs[1] were immobility, incontinence, mental abnormality, falls and strokes. These are all conditions that could have perhaps been cured or at least ameliorated some times many months or even years before the final admission. Sometimes, a single episode of incontinence in an older person leads to immediate panic. Isaacs has commented that those doctors who might be interested in an abnormally functioning heart valve in an old person appear to be disinterested in incontinence caused by a faulty urethral valve, even though the mechanics of the failure are no less delicate and the failure no less disabling.[2] It is not surprising that at the age of 75 a person who has emptied his bladder approximately 175,000 times successfully may sometimes have some accidents, but there is likely to be a reason for these accidents. Sadly, failure of bladder control in old age may immediately lead to medico-social bankruptcy.

How Important Is the Problem of Incontinence in the Elderly?

The Northwick Park Hospital Epidemiology Unit has estimated that 12.5 per cent of women and 7.6 per cent of men over 65 on the lists of general practitioners (and therefore living at home) were incontinent twice or more a month.[3] The survey suggested that well over 15 per cent of men and women were likely to be regularly incontinent over the age of 85 and that urinary incontinence accounted for 80 per cent of the incontinence problems. An important finding was that the prevalence of urinary incontinence known to health and social services prior to the survey was far below that revealed by the survey. There are of course many reasons for the under-reporting of illness in old age and this will be discussed subsequently, but it is surprising that a symptom as distressing as incontinence had not been brought to the attention of family doctors or community nurses.

The problem is even more serious in residential and nursing homes, and in hospitals. A recent survey of elderly people in residential homes managed by the London Borough of Camden revealed that one-quarter of residents were incontinent each day,[4] about a third needed help to go to the lavatory and incontinence was significantly associated with depression as well as with dementia — only one-third of the residents were thought to be free of dementia. The survey revealed a very worrying level of both psychiatric and physical morbidity including incontinence, the latter often being related to the underlying psychiatric disturbance. Willington[5] had previously suggested that the overall incidence of urinary incontinence in old people's residential and nursing homes, and long-stay geriatric and psycho-geriatric wards was between 25 and 50 per cent. It must be commented that the staff in these situations are not necessarily blameless in that they may also just accept the incontinence as inevitable. They may fail to realise that a poor quality environment with distant and inadequate toilet facilities, the provision of chairs and beds that are difficult to get out of, lack of physical and psychological stimulation and the use of drugs that affect mobility, stability, and bladder function may all be potent factors in initiating and maintaining unnecessary incontinence. A recent communication by Tobin and Brocklehurst[6] described the finding that 10 per cent of residents in a large number of local authority homes for the elderly were incontinent of faeces at least once a week. About three-quarters had been incontinent for more than a year and about three-quarters were severely demented. In more than 50 per cent, faecal impaction was the primary cause of secondary incontinence (see also Chapter 4). A follow up survey revealed that two-thirds of the previously incontinent residents were no longer incontinent as a result of appropriate treatment of problems revealed by clinical examination during the first survey.

These figures all suggest that incontinence is a very substantial problem in the elderly. Obviously, nursing and care staff in hospitals and homes must have a major commitment to be educated about and understand the reasons for incontinence and know about the ways of preventing or minimising it, and how to deal with it cleanly, humanely and with dignity if it cannot be prevented. In the community, the figures suggest that a general practitioner with a list of about 2,000 to 2,500 patients is likely to have between 150 and 250 patients suffering from urinary incontinence, most of them being over 65 years old. This highlights the need for appropriate under and postgraduate teaching of doctors about important aspects of geriatric medicine, and also highlights one of the basic criticisms of current medical school curricula which is that they tend to be specific disease-orientated rather than looking at functional disturbance and whole person medicine. It has also been suggested that an energetic, aggressive, and well-informed approach to the problem of incontinence would not only reduce the prevalence of a distressing sympton but be cost effective. It is unlikely that the situation has changed much since Exton-Smith and colleagues[7] showed more than 20 years ago that some 25 per cent of nursing time in a geriatric ward may be spent dealing with incontinent patients. Somewhere between 100 and 200 million incontinence underpads are probably being used yearly in the UK, in hospitals, homes and at home, at an annual cost exceeding £10 million. These are often purchased without regard to quality or the particular needs of individual patients. The choice of an appropriate aid requires skill and a range of available equipment. This obviously highlights the need for better communications between doctors, nurses and suppliers.

Finally, to conclude this section the obvious point must be that the geriatric scenario is one of a predominantly female population. There are about 2 female pensioners for every elderly man, and over 85 the proportion in the UK is 3 to 1. This sex linked survival pattern obviously accentuates a female predisposition to urinary incontinence, compared with men. There is no particular evidence that the female bladder per se is more susceptible to defects such as the irritable detruser syndrome or atony, but the shorter female urethra compared with the male and the post-menopausal oestrogen deficiency may contribute to bladder and perineal weakness.

Ageing and Urinary Tract Dysfunction

Whilst acknowledging that the majority of the incontinence problems in older people are due to a specific cause, ageing, i.e. age related, changes in the structure and function of the genito-urinary tract may be clinically significant. These changes are not apparently due to any specific identifiable disease process although it must be stated that certain uncommon diseases, such as diabetes, do appear to be associated with an increased risk of what might be called accelerated ageing of tissues generally over and above the specific diabetic complications that so commonly affect various organs including the bladder. Ageing or senescent changes in themselves may be coped with as the body generally has very substantial reserves of functional capacity, but when combined with other problems can easily summate and produce incontinence. For instance, hypnotics given to an old person with disturbed sleep may ensure a good night's rest, but at the cost of incontinence by reducing their ability to cope with increased nocturnal urine production and frequency. A urinary tract infection seems to be more likely to precipitate incontinence in older people compared with younger people who can be very ill with symptoms of cystitis or pyelonephritis but are not incontinent. This may be because of changes in bladder and urethral control, combined with a deterioration in the genito-urinary tract epithelium which render it more susceptible to infection and inflammation and may precipitate incontinence. However, incontinence may suddenly develop as a result of an apparently trivial 'insult' even in a previously continent and ostensibly fit old person, who has quietly developed one or more of the ageing changes.

Ageing effects include:

(1) A loss of muscular elasticity in the genito-urinary tract and in the pelvic and abdominal musculature. Although this is included in this list like many of the other changes listed below it may be that there is an identifiable reason for the loss of muscle tone such as atrophy due to underuse, or hormonal deficiency.

(2) A decline in connective and supportive tissue tone, possibly for the same reasons as 1.

(3) Atrophic, so-called 'senile' vaginitis. The adjective senile is only used because it is part of medical terminology but does not mean that any other part of the person is necessarily physically or psychiatrically degenerating. Again, it is believed that this is related to oestrogen lack.

(4) A decreased resistance of the tissues of the urinary tract to infection and injury. Changes 1 to 3 and a systemic reduction in infection responses via the immune system of white cells, antibodies etc. are thought to be responsible.

(5) Changes in the bladder include a reduction in its capacity, and an increase in the likelihood of trabeculation and diverticula developing in the bladder wall especially in older men. There is an increased risk of bladder stones in older people, often associated with infections and of course the calculus may be disposed to infection often with *Proteus* organisms.

(6) An increased risk of neoplasia in the genito-urinary tract, including the prostate gland and colon. This cannot really be regarded as a 'benign' senescent change, but is included because it is likely that

longevity is implicated in the multi-factorial aetiology of malignant disease for a variety of reasons such as the chance of an abnormal cell division occurring, the length of exposure to carcinogenic agents and hormone changes.

(7) Loss of renal tissue even without evidence of specific pathologies such as diabetes, arteriosclerosis, infection or hydronepherosis. There may only be between a quarter and a half of the functional renal tissue left at the age of 70 compared with that present at the age of 25. This change tends to be reflected in a reduced filtration rate, a reduction in the renal urinary concentrating power, a reduction in the total daily urinary output and an altered pattern of urine production with a tendency to increased nocturia. In my own random survey in 1974 of elderly people living in the community almost 50 per cent were frequently getting up at night to micturate twice or more. Only the minority were incontinent, but of course this pattern would predispose some to incontinence particularly if they were on hypnotics, sedatives, or diuretics, or had poor mobility or distant toilets or any combination of these factors.

(8) Benign prostatic hypertrophy in men and the so called syndrome of bladder neck obstruction or fibrosis in women cannot legitimately be described only as senescent changes as they are clearly pathological, but again are included because they may have senescent hormonal and/or degenerative factors in their aetiology. Whether or not the female outlet obstruction syndrome is truly analogous with prostatic hypertrophy is not clear. Histologically, this syndrome may be associated with a change in the bladder neck epithelium from transitional to squamous type, and with interstitial and fibrotic changes including lymphocyte and macrophage infiltration. It is generally agreed that the urethra and trigone are particularly sensitive to the levels of oestrogen. It is suggested that changes in the lower genito-urinary tract may predispose to retrograde infection, and also to the urethral 'syndrome' which may reflect an abacterial cystitis.

(9) The condition of detrusor irritability, the so called unstable bladder, is now generally regarded as a pathological entity, and is relatively common in older people. Its cause is not known, and there may be more than one cause, but it is possible that ageing is a factor. This condition usually progresses through diurnal frequency to nocturnal frequency, followed by urgency and then incontinence. Although it is suggested above that at least part of the changing

pattern of urinary flow in the elderly is due to renal changes, the frequency of nocturia suggests that early detrusor deterioration may also be present in many older people.

(10) The age-related deterioration in the sense of smell affecting so many older people could also be a factor. If there is a lack of awareness of unpleasant smells, social difficulties can arise.

Causes of Urinary Incontinence

Before looking in detail at the main, important causes, it is important to review some other general factors not already mentioned as to why disturbed incontinence is so common as we age.

(1) Many of the pathologies occurring in old age are chronic or only partially reversible.

(2) The symptoms and signs of disease in old age are often modified, or completely non-specific. Accurate diagnosis is difficult and sadly may not even be attempted. The symptoms and signs may be labelled (dismissed) as 'because of old age, and what can you expect'. For instance, infection may not be considered when incontinence develops and the elderly person is not particularly pyrexial, does not have a raised white count, nor abdominal pain to suggest renal involvement.

(3) Individual pathologies in older people are often multi-factorial in their aetiology. Advancing age is likely to be associated with the 'acquisition' of accumulated multiple pathologies. This pathology is often not known to the person's general practitioner. Fifty per cent of disabilities discovered by the survey of Williamson and his colleagues[8] of old people living at home were not previously recognised and half of these were potentially remediable. In a survey in my own department, we found that the average number of problems in inpatients was more than nine. The number would have been even higher if we had separated some of the abnormal and functionally disturbing aspects of individual diseases, e.g. motor impairment, hemianopian, co-ordination and speech problems, and perceptual and body image defects in a stroke victim. It is also common to discover if screening and voluntary tests are carried out that biochemical, haematological and other results are outside the normal range. These changes may not be of any great biological significance, and may return to normal as the

person improves, but they may reveal an unsuspected diagnosis such as thyroid dysfunction, and may specifically indicate a degree of previously unknown renal impairment. Summation of more than one causative factor is, therefore, very likely. For instance, there may be a urinary tract infection, constipation, detrusor instability, diabetes and osteo-arthritis. If in addition a diuretic is given and there are only two toilets for a thirty-bedded ward, incontinence is almost inevitable.

(4) The age-related decline in organ structure and function of kidney, bladder and bowel tone and co-ordination, and of produced organ reserve capacity to cope with pathological insults has already been described. These changes not easily described as diseases in the international classification codes will frequently be part of the incontinence jigsaw.

(5) The iceberg of undiscovered and unreported disability in old age already referred to reflects a lack of awareness of the possibility of accumulated multiple pathology and disability and also probably because society as a group and old people and their carers have low expectations. They may be undemanding and they, their carers and their doctors and nurses may assume that problems such as incontinence are unavoidable or, alternatively, that they should not be asked about or looked for and energetically investigated and treated. At the very least the incontinent patient should be *properly* examined once the fact of incontinence is known to the doctor. It is worrying that in the survey by Williamson and colleagues already referred to that three times as many urinary problems were not known as were known.

Bad 'attitudes' to the elderly sometimes described as ageism, that can in some cases be charitably ascribed to inadequate education of doctors, nurses including health visitors, social workers and others in both the under and postgraduate curricula must be identified as a major part of the problem of incontinence in old age. This may lead to incontinence as well as to a failure to bother to diagnose and treat it. Newman has made some very pertinent comments about attitudes to 'old folks in wet beds' in an Open University publication.[9] He highlights the problems of a change in environment such as admission to hospital and points out that older people are less able to change their normal pattern responses when their environment changes. The environment, particularly in hospital is not only a difficult one in terms of the usually quoted problems of too few nurses, problems of getting over cot sides and distant toilets, the use of many drugs that may predispose to incontinence, but being ill and in hospital often equates with being in bed. Patients in bed often have difficulty micturating and become constipated. 'Bed is bad' is a common geriatric dogma. Newman also points out that admission to an institution may present the old person with such a massive change in the fabric of their normal daily life that a breakdown of normal functions is very likely. Geriatricians are not exempt from criticism, and it is of course all too easy to become interested and enthusiastic about sorting out the problems in the newly admitted old person and neglect the origins of geriatric medicine in the longer-stay wards where incontinence can be a major and protracted problem for patients and nurses.

Newman describes the situation which may often occur in a hospital ward when the nurse preparing for the ward round or the doctors during the ward round discover a wet patch on the bedclothes. Hopefully, if the ward has enough linen the bed will be changed quickly but this is regarded as a nursing problem and may actually be ignored by the doctors. If there has been blood on the bed clothes, it might have been much more likely to provoke interest and action to diagnose and treat the cause. It would have been likely to be fairly easy to investigate and identify and treat the cause of the blood but a wet patch may be ignored by the doctor or only prompt a discussion with the nurses about whether the patient should be catheterised.

Many medical textbooks have little or no reference to incontinence, or if they do they establish and perpetuate myths such as that a stroke or Parkinsonism cause incontinence. Infection is by no means the inevitable cause of incontinence in old people — if most younger people with urinary tract infections are not incontinent even if they have uncomfortable frequency of micturition then why should infection always make old people incontinent? Similarly, by no means all severely demented old people are necessarily incontinent.

It is also an interesting fact and presumably reflects poor attitudes and education, often reinforced by senior doctors, that the label of incontinence in an ill patient, particularly if he or she is elderly, is likely to provoke a stark refusal to find a bed. Even though incontinence may sometimes be due to psychosocial breakdown, stress responses and environmental changes it is just as much a medical problem as more respectable pathologies such as a coronary thrombosis. It is not purely a social problem. It is just as bad for the sufferer as many other medical complaints and should still be treated with respect and medical skill.

If a doctor became incontinent he would be hammering on the door of a neurologist or urologist for immediate attention.

Causes of Urinary Incontinence

Table 6B.1 briefly indicates the substantial list of general problems that may cause urinary incontinence in older people. It will already be clear to the reader that any combination of these problems may be present in the same individual and indeed that this will almost be the rule rather than the exception. There is no entirely satisfactory way of presenting such a large list, but it is a help in trying to sort out the diagnosis by an easy flow chart of diagnostic questions and answers, the so called algorithmic approach. Hamdy[10] broadly divides the causes of urinary incontinence as iatrogenic, pelvic, neurological and others. Another simple approach would be to group causes broadly as intrinsic, local, or general. Another important diagnostic grouping to establish is what the pattern of the incontinence is during the 24 hours and whether it is trivial and occasional or short lived, or frequent and sustained.

Briefly reviewing the causes highlighted in Table 6B.1:

Table 6B.1: Causes of Urinary Incontinence in Older People

'Temporary'

Any acute systemic illness (including urinary tract infection)
Immobility
Cerebrovascular accident
Retention with overflow
Confusion/Dementia
Depression
Incontinent behaviour
Drugs
Changed environment
Inadequate environment

'Permanent'

Virtually all the above causes plus:
Any chronic systemic illness
'Stress' incontinence
Prolapse
Atrophic urethro-vulvo-vaginitis
Unstable bladder
Carcinoma
Calculus

'Temporary' Causes

Just as confusion can occur in a previously mentally normal old person during the course of any *acute systemic illness*, so can urinary incontinence develop. If the person gets better, the incontinence should improve (but of course if a catheter has been used there may be secondary problems perpetuating the incontinence). If an illness continues and becomes chronic, then incontinence may also continue indefinitely.

The problems of *immobility and instability* are closely linked, and may be caused by conditions such as arthritis, Parkinson's disease, stroke, as well as painful musculoskeletal conditions. Weakness from whatever cause may not only immobilise an old person but may produce a vicious circle of disuse, stiffness, pain on movement and muscular weakness. Even if the person is able to get up and walk they may be rather unstable. Even simple 'flu can weaken muscles, affect posture and gait and again lead to postural hypotention and produce a fear of falling.

Immobility does also of course lead to alteration in bowel tone with the likelihood of constipation, and again this may be a factor in producing urinary incontinence. It cannot be emphasised too strongly that immobility is frequently associated with urinary incontinence and this is one of several important reasons why geriatric physicians usually say bed is bad for patients. In one survey, 83 per cent of a group of elderly patients with urinary incontinence were immobile.[11]

Strokes are one of the many important causes of immobility as they often render their victim unable to walk (to the toilet) or to reach and handle a urinal. Sometimes it is difficult to micturate in unfamiliar positions, as when confined to a bed or chair. There may also be problems of co-ordination and perception of normal body image which with speech difficulties add to problems of communication about bladder needs. Stroke patients may also be susceptible to infection especially if they have been catheterised, or become constipated, or may have atonic bladders with problems of residual urine. Some patients with a mild stroke have persistent incontinence. This may be because of disturbance of higher cortical control of normal continence. It has been suggested that the inhibitory effect of the cortex on the bladder emptying is reduced as an 'ageing' effect so that some older people may not be able to postpone micturition for more than a few minutes once the bladder starts to fill.[12]

Urinary tract infections are often put first on the list of the causes of incontinence in older people. Anatomical and functional changes in the bladder, urethra, pelvis and the tendency to a reduced resistance to infection in old age are important predisposing factors. Many elderly women may have some residual urine[13] and various diseases such as diabetes may also lead to an atonic neurogenic bladder, the result of which increases the chance of infection. Indwelling catheters are often used in the elderly, to treat the problem of residual urine, to treat retention, as well as managing any incontinence. Sometimes the use of a catheter can mean an elderly person is able to remain in their own home whereas otherwise, unable to manage the incontinence they would be in a long-stay geriatric ward. There is obviously a risk of altering the bladder function and a predisposition to infection.

It must be pointed out, however, that by no means all old people with urinary tract infections are incontinent, nor does the use of a catheter inevitably mean infection and incontinence if and when the catheter is removed. Asymptomatic bacteriuria is often found in catheterised patients and in old people without catheters. Therefore treating the patient with an antibiotic as a result of the laboratory report is not appropriate. As many as one-fifth of women over 65 out of hospital have been found to have bacteriuria, and somewhat surprisingly a similar figure was found in men over 70.[14] It must also be remembered that urinary tract infections may have specific pathological and potentially remediable causes.

The problem of *retention with overflow* may occur in elderly women and men. It may be due to prostatic obstruction, or obstruction caused by constipation or to bladder neck syndrome in women associated with hypertrophy and stricture. Old people are no less likely than younger people to have rare but serious problems affecting the spinal cord such as paraplegia due to trauma, infected lesions, particularly due to primary or secondary malignancy of vertebral bodies. The neurological causes of retention with overflow involve the spinal reflex and atonic neurogenic bladder, the first being due to interruption of the neural connections between the sacral bladder receptors and the cortex, and in this condition reflex emptying occurs whenever the pressure in the bladder reaches a certain level, with involuntary emptying of the bladder. This is distinguished from the situation where there is dysfunction of sensory fibres from the bladder and sacral nerves to the cortex, but some voluntary control is maintained and the patient can sometimes voluntarily start micturition. The bladder becomes distended and overflow or infection may develop. Nerve lesions affecting the lower spinal cord and cauda equina may produce a reflexively autonomous bladder with residual urine associated with frequent uninhibited incontinent emptying.

Confusion from any cause may lead to incontinence but both may also develop from one underlying process such as a urinary tract infection. These symptoms may also be features of almost any illness, which remit if the illness is acute, but may be sustained if it is chronic. Confusion can also be caused by the use of certain drugs as well as a change to an unfamiliar environment, and incontinence may be the consequence of either. Confusion may be treated but cannot be completely alleviated if there is an underlying chronic problem like dementia. However, not all those clinically so labelled are in fact demented. They may have depressive pseudo-dementia.

Depression in old age is often not as clear cut as in younger people and it is very easy to regard slowed up and withdrawn old people as being demented when in fact they are depressed. Incontinence is not synonymous with confusion nor with dementia, but a confused person is often likely to become incontinent. They do not know or care where the toilet is, and cannot find their way there. They are likely to lose the normally acquired acceptable social behaviour of continence, but beware . . . the definition of incontinence is doing the wrong thing in the wrong place at the wrong time, i.e. inappropriate behaviour in place and time. An old person at home may micturate at odd times, and into convenient but unusual receptacles. When they fall ill and are moved somewhere else (and of course may be under the influence of a toxic disease and under the influence of drugs) it is easy to label them as an incontinent dement because they cannot avoid incontinence. They have no way of reproducing their usual pattern of micturition.

Although one cannot emphasise too strongly that incontinence in older people should initially always be regarded as due to some underlying cause, possibly remediable, it is interesting to note that it can sometimes be due to intentional or subconscious *naughty* behaviour. This may be just as reversible as the other causes described, but does not conveniently fit into a traditional differential diagnostic list of diseases.

Firstly, there is the situation Gray and Mackenzie[15] describe of an incontinent sufferer feeling that she has returned to her childhood. Ashamed, and perhaps having scolded her own children when they were incontinent she expects to be scolded herself and may try and hide the fact of her incontinence.

A completely different type of incontinent behaviour occurs in a resident in an old people's home or a patient in a hospital ward where there is an inadequate response to requests for toiletting or no provision of a call aid. Whatever the explanation this lack of attention actually produces incontinence, and this may not be fully realised by the staff.

Finally, particularly in the place where geriatric medicine had its roots, in the long-stay ward, and also in residential and nursing homes, incontinence may be an attention-seeking device. Alternatively, it may reflect boredom, apathy or depression. This may seem surprising to a continent member of staff, but the development of incontinence after admission to a home or hospital may be a behavioural response rather than due to intrinsic physical, obvious psychiatric, or extrinsic environmental factors. The psychological mechanisms of behavioural abnormality include repression, dependency, rebellion, insecurity, attention seeking, disturbed condition reflexes and sensory deprivation. It is important that staff recognise the social and medical aspects of the problem. This can be achieved by education so that staff can be trained to act and respond appropriately.[16]

Iatrogenic causes of incontinence, are, alas all too common. *Drugs* may cause, precipitate, or aggravate existing incontinence. For instance, diuretics can obviously cause urinary incontinence, or like many drugs can cause postural hypotension affecting mobility. As already suggested the various drugs used to affect mood abnormalities and to sedate may produce incontinence, particularly during the night. Anti-cholinergic drugs can cause retention and incontinence as a result of overflow. These drugs include certain anti-depressants, phenothiazines, propantheline, and some drugs used to treat Parkinson's disease. Also, as already pointed out, many drugs can cause confusion which is sometimes associated with incontinence.

Why is there such a Pandora's box of drug problems in the elderly? In brief:

(1) Polypharmacy. Many old people take many drugs, therefore simple arithmetic suggests an increased incidence of toxicity from any one of the drugs, and a greater risk of adverse interactions between them.

(2) Drugs are more likely to cause problems the older their recipient. Metabolic and clearance mechanisms, including renal clearance, deteriorate as a result of disease and senescence.

(3) Drugs are sometimes used incorrectly in the elderly because the diagnosis is not established clearly, and they are sometimes continued

unnecessarily long after the problem they were prescribed for has remitted.

(4) Faulty compliance, i.e. misunderstanding by the patient of the correct regime. This may lead to drug toxicity as well as to ineffective treatment.

It has already been mentioned how confusing it can be for many old people to have a *change of environment*, for example to be moved from their own home or into hospital, particularly if they are ill. It is common to find old people being moved around in a hospital ward or quite often from one ward to another frequently to make room for someone else, whereas their need is to settle down and adjust to a new unchanging environment. Unless they are told and reminded they may also not know where the toilets are or be able to find their way there and back to their bed.

In many homes and hospitals an *inadequate environment* makes continence precarious. Chairs must be easy to get out of, there should be non-slip floors and rails at convenient points, sufficient toilets, and these fitted with simple grab rails to allow a disabled person to see to their own bodily functions. Geriatricians often tell their students to imagine themselves spending a weekend without the use of their right hand and see how they get on with the normal activities of daily living. Old people in hospital are rarely allowed to have a commode by their bed, although they may be used to keeping themselves continent at night by the use of one.

'Permanent' Causes

All the above causes were included in Table 6B.1 as being possible causes of temporary urinary incontinence. Virtually all of them could also lead to more sustained and sometimes permanent incontinence. In addition, any more chronic systemic illness may lead to incontinence by the pathways already described. Anatomical and functional abnormalities of the lower genito-urinary tract may be caused by disease, hormone deficiency, or ageing or, of course, may follow surgery. This may lead to stress incontinence, and prolapse or atrophic urethral-vulvo-vaginitis. It is important to point out that not all people who lose urine when they move or cough or strain are necessarily suffering from stress incontinence. Even if there is evidence of weakness of the pelvic floor they may well also have an unstable bladder. The development of incontinence after surgery for prostatic obstruction whether it is by open operation or a trans-urethral resection may not be due to surgical damage of bladder neck and urethra but because the unstable bladder has now been revealed by the removal of the obstruction. Detrusor irritability may be worsened by drugs such as diuretics, hypnotics and alcohol.

Other causes of urinary incontinence include bladder stones, carcinoma of the bladder and prostate, and cervix or uterus in women, and of the colon in either sex. Urinary incontinence may develop as a result of a fistula developing into the urinary tract by invasion from a colonic carcinoma or diverticulitis.

Surgery for prolapse, or stress incontinence, prostatic disease, or carcinoma can sadly reveal or even cause bladder problems. In one study surgery for genuine stress incontinence appeared to lead to detrusor instability in one-fifth of the patients.[17]

Management of Incontinence

Teamwork

Good geriatric care is about efficient teamwork, i.e. sufficient numbers of well trained and sympathetic professionals and volunteers, equipped with good quality hospitals, residential and sheltered places, day hospitals and day centres, with modern equipment to ensure maximum independence even for the most disabled, with the strongest possible links forged between health and social services. Such services need to be complemented by on-going education of professionals, volunteers, carers and the elderly themselves not only at the national level but it is also very necessary at the local, district or borough level.

Not all incontinent victims are elderly, but the geriatric service is likely to be centrally involved in developing the 'continence promotion team' as recommended in a recent Kings Fund report.[18] Ideally, this will work in and out of hospital by providing:

(1) Diagnostic expertise, e.g. including gynaecological, urological, neurological and geriatric advice backed up with appropriate investigations such as video voiding cystometrography. Sadly, it is the experience in many geriatric departments that urological and gynaecological advice is sometimes not very forthcoming.
(2) Up to date knowledge about, and examples of aids to daily living.
(3) Liaison with social services to help provide incontinent laundry services and facilitate the granting of attendance allowances where appropriate. Even where laundry services exist to help incontinent

patients and their relatives, the infrequency of pick up and delivery of soiled linen and the under provision of spare linen often make the service fall far short of what is actually needed.

Ideally, perhaps, the most effective base for such a team would be in a geriatric day hospital, based in the district general hospital.[19]
Individual team members would include:

(1) Nurses, who would be involved both at home and in hospital, and often one nurse employed as a district continence adviser.
(2) Physiotherapists providing general rehabilitation for various disabilities to ensure maximum mobility, minimal clumsiness and good stability of posture and gait.
(3) Occupational therapists who work to ensure disabled people reach their maximum function potential.
(4) Supplies officers and manufacturers should be valuable allies, when made aware of the needs of patients in terms of incontinence aids.
(5) General practitioners as well as hospital specialists.

Urinary incontinence in old people can often be cured or if it cannot be cured it can often be reduced, i.e. improved, and it can be managed comfortably and hygienically much more often than many doctors, nurses and victims realise. Nearly always it can be made more tolerable. It seems to be very difficult to bridge the education gap between high powered technologically orientated medicine and the provision of educational information at a much more basic level. For instance, there are simple information booklets freely available but not often known about — for example one by Smith and Nephew.[20] This booklet neatly divides incontinence into broad groups of stress, urge, sensory and locomotor problems.

Table 6B.2 attempts to summarise the main approaches to the management of incontinence in older people. Thorough documentation of the history and circumstances of the disturbed continence must be followed by careful examination. Often, investigations will be necessary before deciding on specific treatment(s) or alternatively how best to control the effects of incurable incontinence. Careful observation of the pattern of incontinence, and how the victim responds to treatment, is important, whether it is in the use of antibiotics or the results of a toiletting regime. Eastwood and Warrell[21] have suggested that 'major errors in clinical diagnosis' occur in subjects with stress incontinence. Geriatricians often suggest that detrusor abnormalities should be looked for as they are likely to be a frequent cause of incontinence in the elderly, and can sometimes be misdiagnosed as stress incontinence. It is often assumed that irremediable bladder instability will only respond to appropriate medication. Simple bladder education may be very successful in controlling the situation by helping to restore some cortical control. This is important because drug treatment of the irritable bladder syndrome is rather unrewarding in many older people. Placebo treatment was the most successful in treating 'urge' incontinence in women![22] A leader in the *Lancet*[23] stressed that local treatments of the bladder may be successful, as may be surgical denervation. Another leader in the same issue of the *Lancet*[24] reviews artificial bladder implants, at present a very North American approach, and mentions a relatively high cost − £2,000. This is actually rather low compared with the suffering, and with the cost of long-stay care, catheters, condoms, antibiotics and so on.

Table 6B.2: Approach to Old Age Urinary Incontinence

	Disturbed Continence	
	Diagnosis	
History (from others)	Examination	Investigations

Drugs	General
	Abdominal
	Rectal
	Vaginal
		Urine culture
		Screening blood tests
		Radiology:
		  IVP
		  Cystometrogram
		  Ultrasound

	↓	
	Management	
General Curative	More Specific Curative	Skilful Control if Cure Impossible

Treat Infection
  Constipation
  Immobility
  Depression
  Confusion
Check the need for drugs
Improve morale
Improve environment
	Treat atonic bladder
	  unstable bladder
	  prolapse
	  prostatic disease
	  rectal pathology
		Frequent toiletting
		Continence aids
		Skin care

The algorithmic approach to incontinence has already been mentioned. This is really a simple tabulation of pros and cons, differential diagnostic probabilities, the results of investigations and treatment alternatives. Hilton and Stanton[25] have shown that 60 per cent of invasive investigations can be avoided. Eastwood and Warrell's confirmation of the usefulness of the algorithmic approach has suggested that this approach of trying to avoid investigations is most likely to give errors in the diagnosis of stress incontinence. The next article in the same journal[26] also interestingly makes the point that physiotherapy, i.e. a non-medical and non-surgical treatment, is a safe and effective means of decreasing the symptoms and signs of stress incontinence in older women. Despite the relative cost effectiveness of the algorithmic/ diagnostic flow chart approach for the elderly it should not be a barrier to the use of sophisticated investigations if the result could facilitate management, and sometimes reveal treatable conditions.

Table 6B.2 should be looked at in conjunction with Table 6B.1. The tabulation of a simple management approach to the many possible causes of incontinence in older people draws attention to the need for a good history and a thorough examination. Serial observations of such simple measures such as frequent toileting and response to it are important, particularly in older people. The management of the incontinence will depend on the specific conditions found as indicated in Table 6B.1 and the accompanying text in this and other chapters.

Some special points to remember about the management of the various causes of incontinence in older people are:

(1) They may have more than one cause of incontinence, e.g. immobility plus bladder instability plus urinary tract infection. Improving one may be all that is needed to restore continence, or incontinence may only be reversed if all the causative factors are dealt with.

(2) Whilst the urinary incontinence may be the major problem and must be tackled, it may only be part of a complex diagnostic and management jigsaw. It is a socially unpleasant symptom and sign but it may be that other important physical and psychological problems are just as important to treat if the person is to regain maximum health.

(3) Chronically disabled (elderly) patients and those requiring 'terminal care' are a special group. They are likely to have problems of morale, of bladder and bowel function, of skin and deeper tissues at pressure points and to be a strain for carers in their own homes, or to be admitted to homes or hospitals.

There is now substantial, helpful, literature regarding treatment of these groups of patients and their incontinence (see Suggested Further Reading). These various books deal with such topics as the organisation of geriatric services, nursing skills, equipment, education for long-stay patients, therapy in its widest sense for terminal cancer patients and their carers.

Pain relief is only one of the many therapeutic needs in malignant disease. In Cartwright's survey of needs and care of the last year of life in cancer victims,[27] one-third of the subjects had disturbed bladder control, and more than a quarter had disturbed bowel control, 16 per cent had pressure sores. Incontinence and pressure sores were described as very distressing in 50 per cent of those who suffered from them. Similar terminal care problems are also seen in many disabled old people with strokes, Parkinson's disease and arthritis. The time scale of the care in these cases is likely to be longer than those with cancer.

The problem of effectively managing incurable incontinence in the very disabled is that continuing care of the patient should be individuaally tailored choosing from the whole range of aids available. Even in the very disabled, permanently bed- and chair-bound patient, one should often be able to achieve remarkable relief of the problem of incontinence. The use of long-term catheterisation has already been mentioned as appropriate for some patients.

There is considerable argument about the use of antiseptic cover at the time of catheterisation and at regular, possibly daily intervals in catheterised patients and about the use made of systemic antibiotic therapy. The decision should as always be made on the basis of individual circumstances. If antibiotics are used to treat the ill patient showing clinical and bacteriological evidence of infection, it might also seem justifiable to use antiseptic, bladder wash-outs if there is some evidence of debris in the urine.

Faecal Incontinence

Constipation is almost certainly by far and away the most common underlying problem leading to faecal incontinence. There are many causes of constipation in the elderly with age-related colonic dysfunction, possibly many years use of laxatives and purgatives. Various bowel pathologies including diverticulitis and carcinoma, and immobility are all major underlying causes of constipation. Whatever the dietary, pathological and physiological abnormal functional elements that may predispose to established constipation it often seems to be remarkably difficult to cure. Sometimes regarded as an automatic concomitant of old age, there may be a continuing vicious circle of deterioration with less and less frequent bowel openings. Sometimes associated with painful piles or prolapse, or bleeding, it is often accompanied by the need for increasing doses of bowel stimulants ending up with 'clearance' only being achieved by regular manual evacuation. The diarrhoea which results from the constipation, so called spurious diarrhoea, may be wrongly treated and lead to incontinence.

There are also many other causes of diarrhoea in the elderly which may end up in faecal incontinence. Drugs including medicines bought in the chemist without prescription, iron (which can cause constipation) and antibiotics, may also produce diarrhoea. The gastro-intestinal causes are various types of gastro-enteritis, malabsorption with intestinal hurry proctocolitis, e.g. from diverticulitis or ulcerative colitis, ischaemic colitis, prolapse and neoplasm.

A classical presentation of a neoplasm of the colon is with altered bowel habit when a previously normal person develops episodes of constipation, diarrhoea and sometimes faecal incontinence.

Neurological damage to normal colonic control may arise as a result of autonomic neuropathy, e.g. in a diabetic. It also seems that some old people with a so-called magacolon (i.e. a bowel that is grossly pathologically enlarged as is seen in children with Hirschprung's disease) have in fact acquired a pathologically abnormal defect of colonic sensation and muscular control. Another cause of incontinence is of course dementia, but again it must be pointed out that potentially reversible confusion associated with faecal incontinence does not automatically mean a diagnosis of dementia.

Faecal incontinence is less common than urinary incontinence but is likely to be even more devastating and lead to urgent request for permanent institutional admission. The approach to diagnosis and management should be as already described with urinary incontinence. An accurate history of bowel and urinary function should be established. A thorough physical examination (including rectal and where necessary vaginal examination), as well as sigmoidoscopy and barium enema if necessary are all important aspects of the diagnostic assessment routine. A simple straight abdominal x-ray may indicate faecal material in ascending, transverse or upper descending colon not apparent on rectal examination. Examination of the patient's psychiatric state may be indicated.

The management of faecal incontinence will depend on the cause or causes. It may require improvement in mobility, reduction of constipation, treatment of piles and the avoidance of constipating drugs such as analgesics. Surgery for rectal prolapse is even possible for patients at a very advanced age sometimes with remarkable results.

In the longer-term preventive approach, it is interesting to speculate what effect public education might have in persuading people to take more note of the fibre content of their diet both when young and old, so reducing the widespread use of laxatives thought to be a 'good idea'. This together with attempting to maintain mobility in old age, may affect the epidemic of constipation and the complication of faecal incontinence.

Conclusion

Baroness Trumpington said in the House of Lords in 1981[28] that 'Most of these techniques — i.e. for investigation and treatment — and some of the recent major advances in the drug management of urinary incontinence have been known for at least ten years.' She also pointed out that at a London teaching hospital with a specialised incontinence clinic 'only 5 per cent of older patients with established incontinence had ever had the condition medically investigated . . . it is often wrongly accepted as part of the ageing process, not meriting further consideration . . . with little attention to investigation, cure, and management and advice, few elderly sufferers are helped constructively'. She remarked there had been major advances in the treatment of many other conditions such as heart disease and Parkinsonism and found it inconceivable that major advances would not have been made in the treatment of incontinence by concerted research.

Notes

1. Isaacs, B., Livingstone, M. and Neville, Y. (1972), *Survival of the Unfittest: a Study of Geriatric Patients in Glasgow* (Routledge & Kegan Paul, London).
2. Isaacs, B. (1981) in Arie, T. (ed.), *Health Care of the Elderly* (Croom Helm, London), 231-2.
3. Thomas, T., Plymat, K., Blannin, J. and Meade, T.W. (1980), 'Prevalence of Urinary Incontinence', *Brit. Med. J., 281 (2)*, 1243.
4. Mann, A.H. (1984), 'Psychiatric Illness in Residential Homes for the Elderly: A Survey in One London Borough', *Age and Ageing, 13*, 257-65.
5. Willington, F.L. (1978), 'Urinary Incontinence and Urgency', *The Practitioner, 220*, 749.
6. Tobin, G.W. and Brocklehurst, J.C. 'Faecal Incontinence in Residential Homes for the Elderly: The Prevalence, Aetiology and Effect of Medical

Intervention', British Geriatrics Society, Dublin 1985 (a 'poster' presentation).
7. Exton-Smith, A.N., Norton, D. and McLaren, R. (1962), *An Investigation of Geriatric Nursing Problems in Hospital* (Churchill Livingstone, Edinburgh).
8. Williamson, J., Stokes, I.H., Gray, S., Fisher, M. and Smith, A. (1964), 'Old People at Home: Their Unreported Needs', *Lancet 1*, 1117-20.
9. Newman, J.L. (1978), 'Old Folks in Wet Beds', Ch. 29 in Carver, V. and Liddiard, P. (eds.) *An Ageing Population* (Hodder and Stoughton, Sevenoaks), 259-65.
10. Hamdy, R.C. (1984), 'Urinary Incontinence' in *Geriatric Medicine, A Problem-Orientated Approach* (Bailliere Tindall, London), 138-49.
11. Isaacs, B. and Walkey, F. (1964), 'A Survey of Incontinence in Elderly Hospital Patients', *Gerontologia Clinica*, *6*, 367.
12. Exton-Smith, A.N. and Overstall, P.W. (1979), *Geriatrics*, Guidelines in Medicine (MTP Press, Lancaster).
13. Brocklehurst, J.C. and Dillane, J.B. (1967), 'Studies of the Female Bladder in Old Age. Micturating Cystograms in Incontinent Women', *Gerontologia Clinica*, *9*, 47.
14. Brocklehurst, J.C., Dillane, J.G., Griffiths, L. and Fry, J. (1968), 'The Prevalence and Symptomatology of Urinary Infection in an Aged Population', *Gerontologia Clinica*, *10*, 242.
15. Muir Gray, J.A. and McKenzie, Heather (1980), *Take Care of Your Elderly Relative* (George Allen & Unwin, London and Beaconsfield).
16. Jones, S. (1983), 'Education and Life in the Continuing-Care Ward' in Denham, M.J. (ed.), *Care of the Long Stay Elderly Patient* (Croom Helm, London), 122-47.
17. Cardozo, L.D., Stanton, S.L. and Williams, J.E. (1979), 'Detrusor Instability Following Surgery for Genuine Stress Incontinence', *Brit. J. Urol.*, *51*, 204-7.
18. Kings Fund (1983), 'Action on Incontinence', Kings Fund Project Paper, no. 43.
19. Brocklehurst, J.C. and Tucker, J.S. (1980), *Progress in Geriatric Day Care* (Kings Fund, London).
20. Smith and Nephew (1979), *Incontinence*.
21. Eastwood, H.D.M. and Warrell, R. (1984), 'Urinary Incontinence in the Elderly Female: Prediction in Diagnosis and Outcome of Management', *Age and Ageing*, *13*, 230-4.
22. Meyhoff, H.H., Gerstenberg, T.C. and Nordling, J.P. (1983), 'Placebo — the Drug of Choice in Female Motor Urge Incontinence?', *Brit. J. Urol.*, *55*, 34-7.
23. *Lancet* (May 1983), 'Pills for Urge Incontinence', 1080.
24. *Lancet* (July 1983), 'Artificial Bladder Sphincters', 86.
25. Hilton, P. and Stanton, S.L. (1981), 'Algorithmic Method for Assessing Urinary Incontinence in Elderly Women', *Brit. Med. J.*, *282*, 940-2.
26. Castleden, C.M., Duffin, H.M. and Mitchell, E.P. (1984), 'The Effect of Physiotherapy on Stress Incontinence', *Age and Ageing*, *13*, 235-7.
27. Cartwright, A., Hockey, L. and Anderson, J.L. (1973), *Life Before Death, Social Studies in Medical Care* (Routledge & Kegan Paul, London).
28. Trumpington, Baroness (1981), *Hansard* (House of Lords), no. 1130, 125-9.

Suggested Further Reading

Brocklehurst, J.C. (1978), *Textbook of Geriatric Medicine and Gerontology*, 2nd edn (Churchill Livingstone, Edinburgh).

Caird, F.I., Kennedy, R.D. and Williams, B.O. (1983), *Practical Rehabilitation of the Elderly* (Pitman, Tunbridge Wells).

Coni, N., Davison, W. and Webster, S. (1980), *Lecture Notes on Geriatrics*, 2nd edn (Blackwell Scientific Publications, Oxford).

Kratz, C.R. (1978), *Care of the Long-Term Sick in the Community* (Churchill Livingstone, Edinburgh).

Pitt, B. (1982), *Psychogeriatrics, An Introduction to the Psychiatry of Old Age*, 2nd edn (Churchill Livingstone, Edinburgh).

Saunders, C.M. (1978), The Management of Malignant Disease Series, *1 The Management of Terminal Disease* (Edward Arnold, London).

Skeet, M. (1982), *The Third Age, A Guide for Elderly People, Their Families and Friends* (Darton, Longman and Todd, London).

Small, G.W. (ed.) (1982), 'The Dementia Syndrome' in Occasional Survey, *Lancet* (December).

Twycross, R.G. and Lack, S.A. (1984), *Therapeutics in Terminal Cancer* (Pitman, London).

7 INCONTINENCE IN THE COMMUNITY

J.A. Muir Gray

The Community Approach

Few words have been abused more often in recent years than the word 'community'. Community care and institutional care are not two mutually exclusive entities; the institution, whether it is a hospital or an old people's home, is part of the community and the services offered by institutions are community services, no matter how large or technologically sophisticated the institution may be. In this chapter I will discuss the problem of incontinence as it occurs in the home of the affected person and in that sense will be working within the conventional meaning of the word 'community', but do so in the knowledge that other contributors to this book are discussing the problem as it is seen in hospitals and residential old people's homes – the whole of this book relates to incontinence in the community even though much of it concerns the management of the problem in hospital.

There are certain serious problems, such as fractures, which always receive medical attention, but a problem like incontinence which is not so obvious or life-threatening may remain hidden from the professionals who only see a proportion of the people who are affected. This is called the iceberg phenomenon, and the professionals only see the tip of the iceberg (see Chapter 14). Incontinence is a common problem but it is often a hidden problem, which must be searched out before it can be tackled.

Revealing the Hidden Problems

Hidden cases may be considered as being of two types – those in which the incontinence is hidden from everyone and those in which it is known to some people but not to the appropriate professionals.

Where it is hidden from everyone it can often be suspected by the smell in the house. It can be completely concealed, but there may be obvious clues such as soiled sheets hidden in the foot of wardrobes, soiled underclothes hidden in the larder, or newspapers lying in various places on the carpet. If the person lives with other people or receives home help it is usually uncovered fairly quickly but living alone such material may accumulate until the whole house smells.

It is appropriate at this point to consider why incontinence is so often a hidden problem, because an understanding of the reasons for its concealment helps the professional to enable the affected person to admit that he or she is incontinent and to ask for help. The reasons are numerous and complex but, for the purposes of discussion, can be grouped under three headings — hopelessness, shame, and fear.

Hopelessness is a feeling experienced by many disabled people. Suffering from disabling conditions which they know to be incurable and faced by interminable impairment of their abilities, they do not have the prospect of cure or recovery to give them the hope which those who are suffering from treatable disorders enjoy. Some recognise and express their hopelessness and the resulting depression; others convert it into anger and bitterness; and yet others accept a mood of philosophical resignation, of being happy with what they have, and grateful for what is done for them. Those who are hopeless and resigned too often prefer the discomfort with which they are familiar to the possibility of disappointment if they allow their hopes to be raised by the prospect of some amelioration of their condition. This type of response is most eloquently described in Turgenev's short story *The Living Relic*, written in 1874, but still very relevant and useful. The narrator is speaking to Lukeria, who is severely disabled:

'And you can't do anything except lie here?' I again inquired. 'This is the seventh year, master, that I've been lying like this. When it's summer I lie here, in this wattle hut, and when it begins to get cold — then they move me into a room next to the bath-house. So I lie there too.'
'Aren't you bored, my poor Lukeria, don't you feel frightened?' 'What's a person to do? I don't want to pretend — at first, yes, I felt very low, but afterwards I grew used to it, I learned to be patient — now it's nothing. Others are much worse off.'
'How do you mean?'
'Some haven't even got a home! And others are blind or dumb! I can see perfectly, praise be to God, and I can hear everything, every little thing. If there's a mole digging underground, I can hear it. And I can smell every scent, it doesn't matter how faint it is.'
'Listen, Lukeria,' I began finally, 'Listen to what I want to propose to you. Would you like it if I arranged for you to be taken to a hospital, a good town hospital? Who knows, but maybe they can

still cure you? At least you won't be by yourself . . .'
Lukeria raised her brows ever so slightly.
'Oh no, master,' she said in an agitated whisper, 'Don't send me to a hospital, let me alone.'[1]

This attitude is often particularly marked among elderly people who fail to appreciate that their incontinence may be caused by a condition which can be corrected, because they assume that all their disabilities result from the intractable process of ageing.

Shame is felt by many people who are incontinent, a shame not just due to the fact that they have behaved in a manner acceptable only in the early years of childhood but for much deeper reasons. The person who is incontinent has lost control, and loss of control — a cause for severe censure in our society — is both frightening and threatening: consider the attitudes towards people suffering from epilepsy. In addition, the type of bodily function over which control is lost, the excretory function, is one which is particularly upsetting to other people. A bodily substance which is taboo is spread indiscriminately and an act which should only be performed in private becomes public. Every society develops elaborate rules for the control of pollution, as Mary Douglas brilliantly describes in her book *Purity and Danger*[2] but the incontinent person breaks the rules. Of course it can be argued that incontinence is not usually the person's fault, that it is not simply a loss of control but a loss of the ability to control bladder and bowel evacuation, which is very different, but the word incontinence implies that the person has lost control. The Oxford English Dictionary defines it as a 'want of continence or self-restraint. With reference to the bodily appetites especially the sexual passions.' The medical definitions are also given in the dictionary and although they are of ancient origin (Pliny mentioned *incontinentia urinae*), the usage of the word in the last 500 years has implication of weakness and immorality and these remain in the collective unconsciousness of our society.

Fear is a natural response to any departure from normal body function — fear of death or pain, for example. Fear usually motivates people to seek professional help, but elderly people frequently have another fear which leads them to hide the development of disabling symptoms — fear of being obliged to accept institutional care. Their fears and worries of not being able to manage independently are often reinforced by their families, friends and, less often, by the professionals, who exhort them to 'go into a home to be looked after' (see Chapter 13).

These obstacles are difficult to overcome. Education of the public could help reduce the feeling of hopelessness by informing those who suffer and, equally important, their relatives and friends, that the problem of incontinence can almost always be mitigated, and can sometimes be cured, but the feeling of shame which prevents people from seeking help is not easy to dispel. The very nature of the problem inhibits educational efforts — it will be a long time before the producers of television soap-operas feel they can introduce this topic in the way that they have introduced more serious, but now less taboo, themes, such as adultery. Only professionals can overcome the feeling of fear. They must be aware of its existence and sensitive to the sort of people most likely to experience it. If it is stated plainly to the person being visited that 'I'm interested in helping you live on in your own home, if that's what you want to do', then he or she may be reassured and develop enough confidence to discuss the problem freely.

Barriers to communication could be reduced if professionals were more aware of the biases — their own and those of their clients — which always influence the information elicited in interviews. Good professionals are not objective; they are people who are aware of their own attitudes and values, and the biases which these impart to their approach to problems. Social work training concentrates on this; vocational training for general practice is also recognising the need for this type of preparation, but the truth remains that all professionals could be better prepared for interviewing elderly and disabled people — in part by being more aware of *their* attitudes and values and in part, and this is equally important, by being more aware of *the client/patient's* own attitudes and values. This, however, is a matter which can only be improved by better initial and post-qualifying professional education. It does appear that professionals are being better informed about incontinence, but many are still woefully ignorant about the skills and resources of colleagues in other disciplines and services, and this area could easily be strengthened by seminars arranged at local level to bring together all who are interested in working together to tackle the problem.

Psychological Effects of Environmentally-caused Incontinence

The psychological consequences of becoming incontinent are, as we have discussed, severe and serious, but there are additional problems when the incontinence is not caused by internal disorders or diseases but by external factors, i.e. environmental barriers. Incontinence is particularly frustrating for a person who has warning that he needs to go to the toilet, who is aware of the steps which he could take to prevent himself becoming incontinent but is unable to take these steps because some object or person prevents him. No one phsyically stands in his way, but by not appearing to help him when help is needed other people make such a person incontinent just as effectively as if they were barring his passage. The contribution which hospital staff can make to the prevention, or causation, of incontinence is described elsewhere in this book but the same types of problem occur in the community (see Chapter 8).

The person who waits and holds his bladder and bowels until the district nurse arrives at nine o'clock may be terribly distressed if she is no more than a few minutes late and may be unable to hold on much past the time at which relief was expected. Of course all community staff realise how accurately the time of their arrival is measured, how worrying for the immobile person even the briefest period of lateness can be, and do their utmost to keep the time; an objective virtually impossible to achieve in view of the exigencies of work outside hospital. Nevertheless it is easy to underestimate how disturbing it must be to have the time at which one passes water or empties one's bowels determined by others. Perhaps the audience at every seminar on incontinence should be kept sitting for an unspecified length of time before they are allowed to go to the toilet, to bring this message home. If the audience were to be kept in suspense, not knowing whether it was to be two hours, or five or even more before they were to be allowed to relieve themselves they might have a more sensitive appreciation of the feelings of dread and apprehension of those people who are at risk of being incontinent because they are trapped in their room or chair until released by other people over whom they have little authority. No one has described these feelings better than the writer Alexander Solzhenitsyn: although he writes of the plight of those who are held captive by lock and key, those who are held captive by a disabling disease must experience the same feelings:

> But there's not that much to laugh at. We are dealing with that crude necessity which it is considered unsuitable to refer to in literature (although there, too, it has been said, with immortal adroitness: 'Blessed is he who early in the morning . . .'). This allegedly natural start of the prison day sets a trap for the prisoner that would grip him all day, a trap for his spirit — which was what hurt. Given the lack of physical activity in prison, and the meagre food and the

muscular relaxation of sleep, a person was just not able to square accounts with nature immediately after rising. Then they quickly returned you to the cell and locked you up — until 6.0 p.m., or, in some prisons, until morning. At that point, you would start to get worried and worked up by the approach of the daytime interrogation period and the events of the day itself, and you would be loading yourself up with your bread ration and water and gruel, but no one was going to let you visit that glorious accommodation again, easy access to which free people are incapable of appreciating. This debilitating, banal need could make itself felt day after day shortly after the morning toilet trip and would then torment you the whole day long, oppress you, rob you of the inclination to talk, read, think, and even of any desire to eat the meagre food.[3]

Disability and Handicap

The survey by Amelia Harris, *Handicapped and Impaired in Great Britain*[4] emphasised and publicised the need to distinguish between the term 'disability' and the term 'handicap' which is a semantic difference of great importance to everyone meeting people suffering from incontinence whether in their own homes, the houses of relatives, old people's homes or hospitals. The definitions used for the purpose of the study were that disability is the change in physical condition caused by disease whereas handicap is the change in social condition which is caused by the environment. For example, a lady with osteoarthritis of both hips who has impairment of movement of both her hip joints and is unable to climb or descend stairs is severely disabled. If she lives in an old person's bungalow, she can reach toilet, bathroom and kitchen independently. She will not be handicapped in using the toilet or bathroom, but if she lives in a room in a multi-occupied house with toilet and bathroom twelve steps above her and the communal kitchen ten steps below she will be handicapped in reaching the toilet, bathroom and kitchen. This principle is vividly illustrated by a case in which incontinence was cured by a screwdriver:

> Mrs A had moved into a purpose-built elderly person's bungalow and was delighted with the results of her move — 'except for the incontinence'. She said to her doctor that she had been incontinent ever since she had moved in, and showed him the reason. Severely disabled by arthritis, she could only walk slowly with a zimmer frame. When

she felt the urge to pass water she had to rise from her chair and shuffle from the living room across the hall to the bathroom. The bathroom door was hung on the side of the door-set beside the right-hand wall and the toilet was behind the open door, fixed to the plumbing which ran along the left-hand wall. Mrs A had to shuffle into the middle of the bathroom, stop, twist her body round without moving her feet, and push the door shut before she could reverse to sit down on the toilet, and by the time she had completed these manoeuvres she was incontinent − 'by the time I get there I've been!' Mrs A suffered from arthritis and urgency and the length of the journey was too great. The doctor· and the occupational therapist phoned the housing department and suggested that the door be hung on the other side of the door-set, beside the wall, thus allowing immediate access to the toilet, but were told politely but firmly, that the design was correct. The doctor told the housing department that he would remove the door himself, for Mrs A, who lived alone, had said she would rather be without a door and continent than have privacy and incontinence. The housing department said that this would provoke a strike; a carpenter was sent round, who removed the door, and also Mrs A's incontinence.

The importance of this distinction between handicap and disability is that it highlights the need to approach the problem of incontinence in two complementary ways: to assess the relative importance of intrinsic factors, namely physical and mental disabilities, and extrinsic factors, namely the design and layout of the environment. The emphasis of this book is, rightly, on intrinsic factors for it is of prime importance to seek out and remedy any underlying physical or mental cause; the emphasis of this chapter is on the extrinsic factors. Even with the most thorough assessment and treatment of their disabilities, some people are still unable to reach the toilet in time. We are concerned with the assessment and solution of environmental obstacles to continence, and thus with the prevention and cure of environmental incontinence.

Overcoming the Handicap

Even after the most careful investigation and treatment some people still remain unable to reach the toilet in time even though they are aware of the need to urinate or defecate. In this type of case it is necessary to try to adapt the person's environment. The professional should ask himself three questions.

1. Can Mobility be Sufficiently Improved to Allow the Person to Reach the Toilet in Time?

The approach to this problem can be summarised in three supplementary questions:

(1) Is chiropody required?
(2) Is there any underlying medical condition, such as arthritis or Parkinson's disease, which is slowing walking speed or makes the person very unsteady?
(3) Would mobility problems benefit from the advice of a physiotherapist?

The provision of chiropody is, of course, difficult to arrange in many areas because of the shortage of chiropodists in the health service, and it may be necessary to arrange for private chiropody with a State Registered Chiropodist. The assessment and advice of a physiotherapist can help with immobilising conditions as well as restoring confidence to those whose balance is impaired, but the provision of walking aids and re-arrangement of the furniture may also be necessary.

If the person is still incontinent after mobility has been increased to its maximum potential the next question which has to be asked is:

2. Can the Journey to the Toilet be Made Easier?

A number of environmental modifications can make the journey to the toilet easier and therefore quicker, and the following supplementary questions should be asked:

(1) Can the person be helped to rise from the chair more quickly?
(2) Will a second banister make the stairs easier, safer, and quicker to climb?
(3) Is a stairlift necessary?

If a physiotherapist (either hospital or domicilary) is not involved, the key person is the domiciliary occupational therapist who can be contacted via the social services department. The therapist's first step will be to try to teach the disabled person a new way of using the environment. If precious seconds are lost struggling to rise from a low 'easy' chair, she may be able to teach them how to move to the front edge, place the feet and hands correctly and move easily and less painfully.

If this fails, blocks under the castors can elevate the chair; and if this fails, a different chair may be the answer.[5, 6]

Similarly, the occupational therapist will ask herself if ascent of the stairs can be made easier by additional rails or even a stairlift. However, unless it is necessary to use other rooms upstairs, this may not be the most appropriate solution, and the alternative of installing a toilet and bathroom on the ground floor can be considered. The third question to ask is therefore:

3. Can the Toilet be Brought Nearer to the Disabled Person?

If a dwelling has no inside toilet, a house renovation grant can be obtained from the local authority. Such a grant covers no more than 50 per cent of the cost of the work, except in certain designated improvement areas, but the local authority has the power to make a maturity loan to cover the rest of the cost of the work, the interest on which, charged at the option mortgage rate, can be paid by the Supplementary Benefits Commission provided that the person is eligible for supplementary benefit (see either Social Security leaflet SB1 *Cash Help from Supplementary Benefit* or leaflet HB1 *Help for Handicapped People*). Although house renovation grants are usually given only to people who agree to improve the whole dwelling, the local authority has the power to suspend these regulations for a disabled person and grant aid for only one piece of work, such as the installation of a toilet. Grants can also be given to landlords, and although house improvement may result in a rent increase, it should not be considered to be inappropriate solely on this account, because a tenant whose income is low, as the income of many a disabled person is, can claim a higher rent allowance if the rent is increased. Local authority tenants who do not have an inside toilet should approach the housing department.

The person to approach for advice is the environmental health officer. Environmental health departments have a wide range of housing responsibilities, particularly in the owner-occupied and privately-rented sectors, and many are very experienced in dealing with elderly and disabled people with housing problems. If the house renovation grant is for a disabled person, it is wise for the domiciliary occupational therapist to be involved in the design of the toilet or bathroom for which grant application is made. Disabled people have to be reminded that they should not undertake or commit themselves to any expense before receiving the local authority's approval that the work has been approved for a grant.

In dwellings in which there is a toilet and bathroom that are inaccessible because of the inhabitant's disability, local authorities can also give financial assistance by means of grants and loans but in this type of case it is more appropriate to approach a domiciliary occupational therapist in the first instance and allow her to co-ordinate the various steps required, steps recently revised and modified in the Department of Environment Circular 59/78 *Adaptations of Housing for People who are Physically Handicapped*. Such modfications, for example the installation of a second toilet and shower at ground floor level, may result in an increase in the rateable value of the house but the Rating *(Disabled Persons)* Act of 1978 laid down that any additional features in a dwelling which were there to meet the needs of a disabled person should qualify for rebate or relief, as described in the Department of the Environment leaflet *Rate Relief for Disabled Persons*. This leaflet and advice are obtainable from the rates department of the council or from the domiciliary occupational therapist.

The Prevention of Environmental Incontinence

The measures described so far have covered the ways in which the handicap of incontinence — that is, incontinence caused or aggravated by the environment — may be overcome. What is even more important is the prevention of handicap by the correct design of the environment in the first instance.

Housing design is for the average person and has one serious defect: many people are weaker or poorer than average. In particular, those who are not only weak and poor, but also severely disabled, have severe and often insuperable environmental difficulties.

If houses and public buildings, furniture and appliances were designed so that everyone, including the disabled, could use them (apart from those with severe disability) then the average person would be able to use them easily. This approach, which would help many disabled people, is not different or special but functional. It could be adopted easily and cheaply and the result is not immediately obvious as being for 'the handicapped'.[7,8]

The most important example in Britain is Mobility Housing which was introduced by the Department of the Environment Circular 74/74, *Housing for Physically Disabled People*. It has nothing to do with mobile homes; the adjective 'mobility' is used to signify that the design has been developed with the objective of facilitating mobility at the entrances and within the dwelling and the design has important features:

(1) Entrances to the dwelling are to be accessible to people who use wheelchairs.
(2) Internal planning should allow for easy movement by ambulant disabled people; including those who use wheelchairs within their homes but are not totally chairbound.
(3) The bathroom, WC and at least one bedroom must be at entrance level.
(4) Door-sets (door frames) should be 900 mm (35″) wide where possible; a door-set of this width allows most wheelchairs to pass through.
(5) Electric sockets should be at the height of door handles.

Mobility Housing will not meet the needs of all disabled people. Those who must live in their wheelchairs require Wheelchair Housing which has many special features, among the most important of which are:

(1) higher space standards;
(2) passage ways 1700 mm (67″) wide and all door-sets 900 mm (35½″) wide;
(3) space around the toilet to allow either frontal, oblique or lateral transfer from the wheelchair;
(4) deferrment of fixing of the toilet bowl until the particular tenant who is to occupy a wheelchair dwelling is known; and
(5) allowance made at the design stage for the fixing of support rails on either side of the toilet, although these should not be fitted until the needs of the individual are known.

The principles behind and practical details of Mobility and Wheelchair Housing are clearly set out in two occasional papers from the Department of the Environment's Housing Development Directorate.[9,10]

The needs of disabled people outside the home have also to be considered, and suitably-designed public conveniences can be provided by all local authorities and managers of buildings used by the general public if they are sensitive to the need. The necessary design features are similar whether the WC is provided as an isolated public convenience or whether it is provided within a large building, and although the guidance given in the Ministry of Housing and Local Government Circular 33/68 *Design of Public Conveniences with Facilities for the Disabled* is currently being revised, this circular still provides a sound foundation for architects.

Health and social services staff have a key part to play in

environmental design as they are the people who are most closely in touch with those who would benefit and can indicate the extent of need. Housing managers, architects and surveyors are able to mobilise the necessary financial resources and have the professional skills to provide such facilities, but unless they are made aware of the need they will be uncertain as to how to use their skills and resources. In too many areas a huge gap still yawns between the health and social services on the one hand and the environmental services on the other, with the domiciliary occupational therapist trying uncomfortably to straddle the gap. No opportunity should be lost to bring together those who work in all these services, to co-ordinate and reinforce the common objective: the prevention and cure of incontinence.

Notes

1. Turgenev, I. (1874), *Sketches from a Hunter's Album* (Penguin Classics edn, Harmondsworth, 1967), 215-6.
2. Douglas, M. (1966), *Purity and Danger* (Routledge & Kegan Paul, London).
3. Solzhenitsyn, A. (1973), *The Gulag Archipelago*, Volume 1 (Fontana, London), 204-5.
4. Harris, A. (1971), *Handicapped and Impaired in Great Britain* (HMSO, London).
5. Hawker, M. (1974), *Geriatrics for Physiotherapists and the Allied Professions* (Faber & Faber, London).
6. Hawker, M. (1974), *Return to Mobility* (Chest, Heart and Stroke Association, London).
7. Goldsmith, S. (1977), *Designing for the Disabled*, 3rd edn (Royal Institute of British Architects, London).
8. Penton, J. (1976), *A Handbook of Housing for Disabled People* (Housing Consortium West Group, Southall, London).
9. Goldsmith, S. (1974), 'Mobility Housing', Housing Development Directorate, Occasional Paper 2/74 (reprinted from the *Architects' Journal*, 3 July 1974; Department of the Environment, London).
10. Goldsmith, S. (1975), 'Wheelchair Housing', Housing Development Directorate, Occasional Paper 2/75 (reprinted from the *Architects' Journal*, 25 June 1975; Department of the Environment, London).

8 MANAGEMENT OF THE ELDERLY PATIENT IN THE COMMUNITY

Malcolm Keith Thompson

Introduction

Within the setting of family or general practice, incontinence is encountered in four classes of patient, and most commonly at the extremes of youth and age.

Children with enuresis are seldom easily assessed. It is fortunate, however, that time is on their side and many become dry during investigations and in spite of treatment. It is also true that they can, in the majority of cases, rely upon a fund, albeit a dwindling one, of goodwill and tolerance from parents. In less than one in eight children with nocturnal enuresis is there evidence of organic disease, but they teach their attendant physicians the golden rule that the approach to the incontinent patient is a personal one, and that if we are to get our perspectives right,we must always avoid narrowing the focus of our attentions on to the incontinent state to the exclusion of the wider view which takes in the whole situation of the patient who wets the bed, and cannot help doing it.

In the second group are found those unfortunate young adults with permanent incontinence resulting from nervous disease or spinal injury. These cases are rare, and the diagnosis is firmly established.

From middle age onwards, the effects of multiple or difficult births combined with involutional changes on a variety of pelvic tissues, produce a not inconsiderable group of women with stress incontinence (see Chapters 2 and 3). Even in a society currently given to more open discussion of all aspects of human physiology, concealment of this socially-embarrassing symptom occurs, and it may be detected for the first time in Well Woman Clinics. A diagnosis will determine whether pelvic floor exercises, or surgical intervention, or both, are needed.

In the geriatric field, the symptom of incontinence is now one of the major problems. Not only is the practitioner witnessing an expansion in the size of the elderly population, but it is expected that he has been trained in those principles of geriatric medicine which accord to his work a more hopeful endeavour, so that patients formerly despaired of, or bundled into hospital, may well be managed in their own homes.

It is upon this fourth group that the remainder of this chapter will concentrate (see also Chapters 6A and 6B).

Incontinence Problems of the Elderly Patient in the Community

For social reasons, the full control of micturition (see Chapter 1) demands a series of basic skills involving the ability to:

(1) initiate micturition at a suitable time;
(2) postpone, within limits, the onset of micturition;
(3) perceive the need to urinate well in advance of reflex voiding;
(4) initiate micturition as a voluntary act when the bladder is partially full;
(5) monitor and interrupt micturition already in progress;
(6) postpone reflex bladder emptying during sleep, responding in time to cortical monitoring of a full bladder, and waking when necessary;
(7) identify the places or circumstances where it is socially aceptable to urinate; and
(8) possess the physical mobility and dexterity to assume and maintain body posture during micturition, adjust clothing, and deal with the doors, locks, flushing systems, seats and washing facilities. (For further discussion of these see Chapter 7 and Appendix C.)

What the General Practitioner Can Do

There are few, if any, incontinent patients who cannot be managed at home by their general practitioner and community nurse. Of course, it must be clear that, before any decision is made, plans should be drawn up by both doctor and nurse, and this may be best achieved during a joint visit made early in the undertaking. The fundamental requirements are that the home circumstances are suitable, and that an adequate diagnosis has been made. It is an essential part of professional training that we define our own attitudes and overcome the feeling of distaste for, and rejection of, the patient that might lead to a sense of therapeutic negativism. It is natural that relatives and principal helpers will be favourably influenced by a demonstration of positive and optimistic planning. We should thus try to relate to the patient and form a proper relationship with him, showing tolerance of the situation coupled with an offer of help in doing something about it. This does not, of course, imply any suggestion that the patient should accept his own incontinence, but he might, for instance, be told: 'Don't let it worry you. We have a problem, and you, the nurse and I will get to work on it.'

Emotional Factors

Two main causes give rise to urinary incontinence: loss of control from the cerebral cortex and local disorders of the urinary tract, to which one may add a number of less well-defined emotional causes which can give rise to apparent incontinence. It is in the interaction between the mind of an old person and his or her environment that acute stress and conflict can result in a reversal of established behaviour patterns. Bed-wetting is but one manifestation, and one in which the general practitioner may be most effective in treating. If ignored or unwisely managed, ths situation can form the first step of a dynamic process of regression and increasing dependency, leading to the bed-ridden patient lying like a foetus in a womb of wet bedding.

The whole way of life of many old people is governed by the routine performance of simple repetitive acts developed over years by custom and convenience. The older a person becomes the less easily is he able to adapt to changes in the environment. The tenuous control of micturition (which has for years been taken for granted) becomes very vulnerable to changes in the internal environment, such as feverish illness, or to social changes, either of which produces anomalies in conditioned signals and responses. In modern Western societies it is hard enough, when old and retired, to retain self-respect, and almost impossible if no longer considered a person of consequence. The loss of meaningful relationships and the resulting emotional isolation can lead to apathy and indifference, or even to the display of paradoxical responses towards nurses and attendants. Certainly, urinary incontinence is more frequently encountered in hospitals and institutions for the elderly, but disordered behaviour in old people can be produced at home where they are needlessly 'babied' and assisted in reversion to infantile behaviour. It is in the power of old people to wet the bed as an unconscious expression of resentment, such as might be felt at any undue delay in assistance in using a commode. This is sometimes observed when a frail old mother has become dependent on her daughter, or a young nurse, with whom she enters into a reverse mother-child relationship. The role of emotional dynamics as factors in producing incontinence are subtle and powerful, and it is not without interest to note that many old people who were formerly obsessional and scrupulous about their cleanliness and tidiness, not only mess the bed with urine and faeces, but also as their inhibitions weaken smear the mess about in what seems a disgusting way, and their original drives to make a mess are revealed. The general practitioner is the person best able to evaluate the patient's premorbid personality.

Mobility Problems

The modern general practitioner, with secretarial back-up, may not only have an Age-sex register, but also use Problem-oriented Records and a Disease Index. He may inform himself in other ways of patients with disabilities who can be entered into an At-risk Register so that they can be given increased surveillance.

The assessment of patients with locomotor disease should include the ability to get out of bed, the time taken to reach toilet, and the ability to handle urinary devices. The adjustment of clothing requires skilful flexion and rotation movements of the hands, and it is important to note whether the arthritic patient can bend sufficiently. Tremor is frequently observed in the elderly and should be correctly diagnosed to distinguish Parkinson's syndrome from other neurological conditions.

Home Modifications

This leads us to a consideration of the suitability of the home, and in particular, the toilet arrangements. It is obviously undesirable that in these days elderly people should need to go outside to use the toilet (see Chapter 7). Within the house the toilet should be not more than 12 to 15 paces from the bedroom, for the urge to empty the bladder is often peremptory. The approach should be safe, well-lit and obstacle-free. The door should be wide enough to allow entry when using a walking aid. It is important that the seat should be sufficiently high and should be raised, because muscles which are only just able to raise the body weight may fail shortly after a period of sleep when muscle tone is reduced. Hand rails for extra support may be considered. Finally, allowance must be made for stiff or arthritic shoulders when installing a flushing system, and attention must be paid to the height and type of door handles and to the way the door opens. The presence of a call system creates a sense of confidence.

Diagnosis and Treatment

It is particularly important for the general practitioner to recognise those cases of acute illness accompanied by mental confusion, where the incontinence produced is usually transient and its duration dependent on the speed with which the effects of the underlying disease can be reversed. Among such cases are infections, toxaemias and the side-effects of drugs known to cause confusion or excessive drowsiness, those such as sedatives and tranquillisers must be reviewed, as well as the diuretics given in full dosage to increase the flow of urine. The effects of unaccustomed alcohol in conjunction with drugs must also be taken into account, and in my experience elderly patients on a visit to their children, for instance at Christmas, may be particularly vulnerable in this respect, quite apart from having to cope with a less familiar environment.

The most common cause of incontinence in the elderly is organic brain disease resulting in the production of an uninhibited neurogenic bladder, with frequency and precipitancy (see Chapter 1, p. 22). Cortical damage usually results from vascular disease, and is often accompanied by a stroke in the acute stage, in which incontinence is almost invariably present, but, as the patient recovers full consciousness, he will regain continence depending on the degree of permanent organic damage, and also on his previous mental state. It must be remembered that he may be prevented by aphasic difficulties from asking for a urinal or bed pan, or find mechanical difficulty in managing such devices. Where moderate mental impairment is encountered, incontinence may occur only at night when control of the bladder is further prevented by sleep. The more demented a patient becomes, the less aware he is of being incontinent and the less he will be affected by it. The incontinence that frequently accompanies terminal illness is a manifestation of the failing powers of the body, and can be anticipated, and arrangements made to ameliorate the possible distress for the patient.

Where incontinence is due to local, urological causes, the diagnosis can often be made at the bedside and may lead on to successful treatment. The most common finding is obstruction to urinary flow resulting in subacute retention. The residual urine so formed reduces the functional capacity of the bladder giving rise to overflow phenomena from the hypotonic bladder, often associated with infection. In men this obstruction is almost always due to prostatic hypertrophy. Less common causes are stone and urethral stricture (see Chapter 2).

In female patients, distortion of the bladder neck with resultant sphincteric weakness, often associated with vaginal prolapse, may produce incontinence (see Chapter 3). Many aged women suffer from atrophic vaginitis and urethritis as a result of oestrogen lack. It must be remembered that in some patients the stratified epithelium of the vagina and urethra may extend to the trigone. The red, angry appearance of the epithelium may be assumed to be associated with an abacterial urethritis and possibly trigonitis, with dysuric symptoms, including incontinence.

An important concept that should never be forgotten is the reciprocal action of bowel and bladder and the effect of impacted faeces, producing both urinary and faecal incontinence. The finding of such a degree of constipation must lead the physician to exclude other pathology, such as cancer of the rectum, or myxoedema (see Chapter 4).

The History

The experienced general practitioner, as an informed observer, will take in much on home visits at a glance, for it is usual to see the incontinent patient first at home. If the patient is brought to the practice centre much opportunity would be missed, and a visit by the practice nurse should be requested.

Before taking a history, much can be gained by noting the patient's surroundings. Is he alone? Is he in bed, and, if so, for how long has he been there? Is the room clean and the patient cared for, or does he lie in dirty crumpled sheets and squalor? What, and where, are the toilet facilities: under the bed, next to the bed, upstairs, in the garden, or are they shared? Is there an odour in the room, for this is often a guide to the presence of infection, and the duration of the symptom? What drugs are being taken?

The investigation should be purposeful, and have as its objective the separation of the manageable from the unmanageable aspects. The examination will proceed with an assessment of the patient's mental state. Awareness by the patient of the incontinent state is important, for unawareness will direct the practitioner to consider a confusional state, with or without underlying cerebral failure. It is here that the testimony of the family, or neighbours, may be sought, the type of onset established, and interpersonal relationships revealed. There is no difficulty where the doctor has kept his patient under surveillance, and noted his observations, particularly the drug list. It is the forgotten patient, the new arrival in the district, or the patient who returns from hospital or from a spell with relatives, who poses problems.

The patient who can give his own history can be asked whether his incontinence occurs during the day, or at night only. He can be asked if he has urgency, pain, interruption, or burning. It is important to establish stream patterns, and the voiding habit. Female patients should be asked for their obstetric history. An exploration of emotional and social factors can be both diagnostic and therapeutic, especially when the spouse is present.

The Physical Examination

The physical examination, following a careful history, can enable the problem to be recognised without resorting to laboratory examinations in the majority of cases. It is important to note such signs as tachycardia, blood pressure, fungal infection of nails and skin, oedema, and obesity, as well as those of locomotor disease, such as lower-limb arthritis, or Parkinsonian rigidity. The emphasis should fall on the neurological examination, including fundoscopy, and abdominal palpation and percussion. It is essential to examine the rectum and bladder, and a bimanual examination carried out in the dorsal position gives more information than when either region is examined separately. In thin male subjects it may be possible to detect residual urine in the retro-prostatic pouch; in the female these pelvic examinations should include the vagina. Such examination should be performed despite difficult emotional states or physical disabilities.

The Investigation

The examination of a fresh, clean-voided urine specimen yields more information than almost anything else. It must be realised that while the presence of glucose almost certainly indicates diabetes mellitus, higher renal thresholds in old people may prevent glycosuria occurring at the same blood sugar levels as in younger subjects. Therefore, blood sugar estimation should be requested. Further laboratory tests will include blood counts, electrolytes, acid and alkaline phosphates, calcium, phosphorous and uric acid. It has been shown that the acid phosphatase can rise and remain elevated for several hours following digital palpation of the prostate. Other routine investigations sometimes required are serological tests for syphilis, and chest X-ray.

The role of infection is not easy to establish, nor is the finding of bacteriuria a simple matter of cause and effect (see p. 40). Incontinence is unlikely to be the cause of infection, but the finding of organisms in a clean mid-stream urine often indicates the presence of residual urine, and obstruction. Mid-stream, clean-catch urine cultures are important for initiation and continuation of specific therapy for infection.

Diagnostic Categories

I have found it helpful to construct a mnemonic as a guide to the classification of patients, and I offer it here for what it is worth. For those flexible and able enough to think through the anatomical and physiological pathways freshly each time, it is perhaps a poor thing. But it is now clear that the causes of incontinence are many and often occur in subtle combinations, any integer of which may be the operant cause. Therefore I have evolved a scheme whereby for those with *reversible incontinence* I remember as 'DAMP':

D – *Diuresis*	(Osmotic)	Renal failure
		Hyperglycaemia
		Hypercalcaemia
	(Drugs)	Strong diuretics
		Anticholinergics (retention with overflow)
		Ephedrine
		Sedatives
A – *Atrophy*	Atrophic urethritis/vaginitis	
M – *Mechanical*	Prostate	
	Faecal impaction	
	Pelvic tumour	
	Stone	
	Stress incontinence	
P – *Psychological*		

For those with *irreversible incontinence* I remember 'PISS':

P – *Post-prostatectomy* symptoms
I – *Inhibition* lost over reflex contractions (from cortical centre in frontal lobe)
S – *Spinal* lesions (motor and sensory loss)
S – *Sensation* loss (peripheral and nerve lesions)

Referral

It is clear that there will be instances where the general practitioner will need to refer a patient for further investigation, since treatment must be directed to the primary condition present in the first instance, as well as to secondary effects, of which the most common is infection. It is, therefore, an important responsibility of the general practitioner to choose the correct avenue of referral. Local lesions should be referred to the urologist or gynaecologist. However, this is not always straightforward as the following case history illustrates.

An 81-year-old lady in my practice with frequency and stress incontinence was successfully operated on by the gynaecologist for prolapse. The accompanying urinary infection was successfully treated in hospital, but, on her return home, she continued to have frequency and dysuria by day and night which was threatening her with physical exhaustion since the toilet was down the garden. The urine was again infected and she was returned to the gynaecologist who reported that there was 'no lesion in the pelvis'. A straight X-ray of the abdomen was ordered, and a stone revealed in the bladder; this was successfully removed by the urological surgeon, with complete resolution of the patient's symptoms.

Access to diagnostic radiography is important. Such tests must be used with judgement, and the excretion urogram (IVP) with a post-voiding film is an excellent screening procedure.

It is important that when he refers a patient the general practitioner should give as much information to the consultant as possible. This would include:

Length of symptoms
Type of onset
Fluid intake and urinary output
Presumptive diagnosis plus investigations carried out
The home conditions
Family relationships
Premorbid personality and mental condition

Related disease
·Drug therapy
Reason for referral.

The main reason for specialist referral is to obtain a voiding cystometrogram (VCMG; see Chapters 2 and 3). Apart from patients with
severe handicaps, from stroke or dementia, this investigation provides
further useful information concerning total bladder capacity, volume
at which the desire to void occurs, the response to the stress of coughing,
and intravesical pressure and flow rates. This is particularly useful in
men who remain troubled with incontinence some months after prostatectomy and in forms of unstable and atonic bladder.

The General Practitioner and the Community Nurse

There was a time when the general practitioner, faced with the prospect
of long-term nursing at home, set about organising a team and educating
it. Much of his success in management depended upon his access to
resources and personnel. In modern practice however the nurse is no
longer regarded as the hand-maiden of the doctor. She, or sometimes,
he, is a fellow professional with an advanced training and special skills.
It is very important that both should share a common pool of knowledge
and that they should have similar attitudes towards the objectives of
their joint care. This is now achieved in many, but not all, group
practices, where nurses are in daily contact with the family practitioner
in respect of a defined population. In this situation they should learn
together and also from each other.

Nursing Assessment

Whether the incontinent patient has temporary or established incontinence the problem should be discussed at the earliest stage with the
appropriate nurse (see Chapter 9). It is customary for male nurses to be
available in many areas for the purpose of nursing male patients.
    Whatever the manner by which the linkage is achieved, and this
varies from practice to practice and region to region, the important
thing is that the pathways between professionals should be open, even
if used infrequently. There has been much in the type of training given
to nurses to fit them to work in a way which warrants the use of the
term 'team', with an appropriate division of labour. Therefore, I advocate making the preliminary visit to the patient a *joint* one. On the way

the nurse can be given the medical background and social circumstances and an idea of the patient's attitude to his illness and the context of his personal relationships. The nurse may have been involved with the patient before, and contribute further from her own experience. This joint visit can be used to plan the approach to the problem. For instance, additional equipment may need to be loaned, or the patient's bed brought downstairs into the living room. Doctor and nurse will need to define their roles, the frequency of their visiting and what to expect from the treatment. It is important also that the principal helpers should be seen, and their contribution discussed. They will wish to know how long their nursing commitment will be required and are usually found to be in need of reassurance.

The facilities for washing soiled linen are often inadequate, the helper somewhat frail and unable to make journeys to a launderette burdened with the washing. These problems are anticipated by the experienced nurse, and the general practitioner can rely upon her to manage not only the sick room, but also to recognise eligbility for attendance and heating allowances and supplementary benefits, where these are needed.

The nurse, or the doctor, may need to mobilise further resources for the patient, such as modifications to the home (see Chapter 7). These may vary from simple additions and fittings such as an angled grab-rail, bath boards, and alarm bells, to electric or portable hoists.

The most difficult skill, and one which is always uncertain, is assessing the qualities of members of a family, or neighbours, as helpers. It is foolish and wasteful to erect a system of care at home if it is going to founder in a short time through lack of support.

Principles of Care

It should be explained to the family that though the incontinence may be irreversible, much can be done to ease the patient's problems and those of his attendants. The basic aim is of course to contain the urine.

The first thing the nurse should be asked to do is to chart the times and amounts of urine passed (see Chapter 2). In certain cases the passage of urine can be anticipated or the patient can be kept dry by regular voiding. Where an appliance is to be worn, males fare rather better than females (see Chapter 9). The disadvantages of these devices, where they are required for demented and confused patients, is that the buckles, straps and snappers are interfered with. Similarly, even the balloon type of Foley indwelling catheter can be dislodged.

If a catheter is used, regular irrigation is necessary. Normal saline at a temperature of 110°F (42°C) or 0.2 per cent sodium citrate solution in normal saline can be used as both are readily available and cheap. A short course of two tablets of Septrin twice daily for three days following catheterisation can be given to reduce the incidence of infection which depends more on the presence of residual urine than on the risk of introducing the catheter. Despite such precautions however, chronic infection often results, and the ammoniacal smell of infected urine becomes apparent to all, except the unfortunate patient. Aerosol sprays or Amplex lotion can be used to deal with these odours.

All patients should be encouraged to be mobile. Far too often it is thought convenient to keep the patient in bed. Even the frailest patient can sit in a chair, and whenever possible should be dressed in day clothes. If protection is needed there are absorbent pads and pants available. Kanga pants described in Chapter 9 are so designed to keep the urine well away from the skin.

There are a number of ways by which patients can be encouraged to help themselves. Toilet arrangements may need modifying by resiting, reseating or relighting. Facilities need to be considered if a patient is going to stay away from home. Frankness with relatives about bladder needs, and the provision of a night light and bed commode will overcome many problems.

Many old people have a warm drink before going to bed. Some substances found in cocoa and tea have a diuretic effect, preventing sleep and mental relaxation. For some it is advisable to restrict fluid intake three or four hours preceding sleep.

Many people fail to realise the reciprocal action of the bladder and bowel. The avoidance of constipation is important, so that advice is needed on sufficient fluid, and roughage in the diet, as well as the need for exercise to maintain good tone in the abdominal muscles. If these measures fail then a faecal softener may be advisable.

The use of drugs and their variable results has been discussed in Chapters 2 and 3. Flaxovate (Urispas) appears to be the most favoured of these, but may be combined with anticholinergic drugs, such as propantheline and emepronium bromide. Imipramine and orphenadrine, have also been used with some effect, but it is important to use these drugs with caution because of the risk of precipitating glaucoma.

The use of oestrogens locally is very effective in atrophic urethritis and vaginitis. The application by the patient is often difficult, however, and quinoestradiol (2 mg daily) is an oral preparation which is thought to have a particular action on the bladder. Antibiotics can be given at intervals in rotation, to control odour. Otherwise their function is limited.

It is important that patients should be encouraged to report early for examination, whenever there is a change in the voiding pattern. Dramatic and obvious symptoms such as haematuria, fever and retention receive quick medical attention but gradual change is easily missed, and relentless progression is the rule in untreated lower urinary tract illness.

The loss of urinary control and sexual function as symptoms need not be equated with the 'ravages of old age'. They are just as worthy of investigation and treatment in the old as in the young. The needs of both are the same: maximum activity, emotional security and physical comfort.

9 THE ROLE OF THE NURSE

Angela M. Shepherd and Janet P. Blannin

Introduction

Since the first edition of this book was written, the continence nurse adviser is no longer a figment of the imagination. Despite changing moods in the nursing world there are now a number of nurses whose sole role is as a specialist in the field of urinary incontinence. This development is a result of pressure and encouragement from the medical profession and the lay public but mostly because of a few determined members of the nursing profession who met together with the editor of this book to form the Association of Continence Advisors in 1981. The original group of six has now enlarged and includes physiotherapists, occupational therapists and doctors as well as a solid core of nurses. With a membership of over 600, the Association meets annually to exchange knowledge. As yet there is no agreed job description for the nurse continence adviser to adhere to, and each nurse who is appointed must develop her own format within the existing system, although the Association in March 1985 produced 'Guidelines on the Role of the District Continence Adviser' (see Appendix A).

The Continence Nurse Adviser

Caring for the differing types of disablement associated with incontinence involves many specialities and a continence nursing adviser requires a comprehensive knowledge of the many problems which may arise in her particular field. Expertise is needed in the outpatient department, in the wards and is at its most demanding in the home. An understanding of the many factors which influence the maintenance of continence and prevention of incontinence is of the greatest importance. One of the main priorities of the continence nurse adviser is to help men and women to maintain their independence. Together with the community nurse, she must work to keep or regain the patient's self-respect.

As well as promoting nursing care there are two other important aspects to the role of the adviser; those of teaching and market research.

As a teacher, the scope is unlimited. Up to a few years ago little interest had been taken in the problems of urinary incontinence and even today many attitudes need to be changed. Both the medical and nursing professions are sadly ignorant of the methods of management and of the innumerable aids which are available. Many medical, paramedical and voluntary groups as well as the social services are involved in the care of incontinent people. They too need instruction so that they have insight into the problem and are better able to help. Formal lectures, practical demonstrations and, most informative of all, an in-service training programme, are all effective teaching methods for this subject.

Market research is a new field for nurses but with manufacturers promoting many different products which may be used by the patient, this is an essential part of the role. Not only are the manufacturers anxious to have access to the consumers in person so that they can improve existing products and develop new ideas, but it is essential to have informed opinion so that the most efficient methods for controlling urinary leakage may be produced. As yet there is no single item of protective clothing or an appliance which is appropriate for the majority of people. Too many alternatives are available, and it is most important to have an expert member of the nursing staff who can sit on appropriate committees to offer advice on the purchase of supplies for both hospital and community.

The continence nurse adviser is a specialist whose role is to co-ordinate patient care, teaching and market research. She is able to maintain continuity of care as well as providing expert knowledge by being available to patients, nurses and doctors and others in the community and in the hospital.[1]

Throughout this chapter it has been assumed that both the patient and the nurse continence adviser are female. Urinary incontinence occurs in both men and women, but is more than twice as common in women. The role of the adviser can be undertaken by either male or female nurses. There is a predominance of women in the nursing profession but there are many instances when a male nurse may be at an advantage in this field. It is because of these different aspects that it may be considered necessary to have members of both sexes working together as a team in hospital and in the community.

The Management of Incontinence

The management of urinary incontinence presents a major problem. It is a condition which is no respecter of age but is particularly prevalent amongst the elderly, many of whom are medically unfit. The nurse has an important role and is able to assist and guide the medical profession in the management in many ways. Ideally, she should be at the grassroots, assessing the social, psychological and medical aspects as they first present within the community and giving appropriate advice to the patient at this level. She may become involved only at the point at which the consultant realises he has nothing more to offer and the patient's self-esteem is at its lowest ebb. It is here that a dedicated and knowledgeable nurse is able to help towards maintaining continence and regaining the patient's confidence.

The need for assessment has been stressed in previous chapters (2, 3 and 5). It is as important in the nursing management as in all other types of treatment; not only assessment of bladder dysfunction, but of the individual and her surroundings, whether she is in hospital or at home. With an increasing insight into the need for a nursing service for incontinent people it is recommended that the nurse continence adviser have a team of resource nurses working both in hospital and in the community. These nurses are to be based in health centres, special schools and old people's homes in the community, and in hospital on those wards and departments where incontinence is particularly common.

The resource nurses with a post-basic training are those with a special interest in the patients with incontinence. As well as continuing with their other duties they are able to undertake primary assessment of the patient, to introduce basic methods of management, and are able to refer any problems to the nurse continence adviser (NCA). She, in turn, can keep the resource nurses informed on local policy and procedures, and is responsible for introducing new ideas and equipment. She is also in touch with doctors both in the community and in the hospital.

In our experience, there is no necessity for consultant cover for a nursing outpatient clinic although arrangements must be present for referral should this be necessary. Because of the clinic's independence, people requiring help can be referred from the different specialities, the family doctor, the health visitors and community nurses, or the patient and her relatives can ask for help directly. A clinic may be held within the hospital, using the already trained urology outpatient staff, or in a health centre where the resource nurses see patients referred by their colleagues or the family doctor. A well-trained nurse will realise the extent of her responsibilities and the need for communication with the referring source and with the patient's family doctor, and above all of the importance of documentation and record keeping.

Outpatient Assessment

General Observations. Some of the most important aspects of the patient's problems will emerge almost immediately, for mobility, dexterity, cleanliness and general attitude can be assessed as he or she comes into the room. Discussion will highlight home conditions, family support and which social services have been involved. It will also reveal whether the man or woman is working, what sort of social life he or she has and the degree of independence and his/her mental attitude towards the disability caused by incontinence.

Associated Factors. After general observations have been made the particular problems associated wtih urinary incontinence should be discussed. Is it stress or urge incontinence or a combination of both? Is it an occasional leakage, continuous incontinence or simply post-micturition dribbling? What is the frequency of voiding by day and by night? Is there a diurnal pattern of voiding? Is there a chronic cough, diabetes, or is the patient in early renal or cardiac failure? What drugs are being taken and for what reason? Are there any precipitating factors and what are the possible causes? How far is it to the lavatory and is it upstairs or at the end of the garden? Is a commode or urinal available? If the patient is already using disposable items, what is the source of supply and what are the financial implications? How are these items disposed of? What are the facilities for washing and drying clothing and bedding?

Examination. Having gained the patient's confidence a brief examination is necessary. With the patient on the couch, clothes must be inspected. These can give some indication of the severity of the incontinence as well as confirming the patient's previous comments. If he or she is wearing incontinence aids these must be checked. Abdominal distension should be noted; this may be due to a full bladder, a pelvic tumour (e.g. ovarian cyst) or simply obesity. What is the state of the skin, has a female patient an obvious atrophic vaginitis or a discharge? Vaginal assessment also gives the nurse the opportunity to estimate the function of pelvic floor muscles and, if weak, now is the time to describe the importance of this muscle group in urinary control and to explain the appropriate exercises.

Most nurses know how to examine the anus and perform a rectal examination. A lax anal sphincter may indicate that there is damage which may also affect the urethral sphincter mechanism. Digital examination will detect chronic constipation and faecal retention, relief of which may help urinary control considerably. The male genitalia should be examined with some care. Does the foreskin retract, is there a pinhole urethral meatus or an undiagnosed hypospadias? If the penis has become retracted or if scrotal herniae are present there will be considerable difficulty in fitting an appliance. With the woman, this is the time to assess the accessibility of the urethral meatus should self-catheterisation become the management of choice. A simple flow rate can be helpful in men to eliminate an outflow obstruction. Women are seldom obstructed but estimation of the volume of residual urine immediately after a free void will highlight a silent chronic retention or hypotonic bladder. A C.S.U. (Catheter Specimen of Urine) taken at this time will provide reliable information on a urinary infection. Results of a mid-stream specimen taken from the elderly are notoriously difficult to interpret.

Management. With this full knowlege of the patient and their problems management can be undertaken on a logical basis. Everyone can be helped to some extent and a positive approach at this stage is most important. Sometimes it is the simple things which give greatest relief. Local application of dienoestrol cream or oral hormone therapy prescribed by a medical practitioner can cure a simple but aggravating atrophic vaginitis and urethritis. Pelvic floor exercises can be understood and practised by the most elderly men and women just as well as by young mothers in the puerperium. In our experience successful re-education of this muscle group can prove most effective.

After prostatic surgery many elderly men lose the ability to milk-back into the bladder the few drops of urine remaining in the urethra at the termination of voiding. A few words of explanation will cure this problem for many. Some men find it easier to void to completion by sitting rather than standing. In others it will help if they are shown how to push the remaining drops of urine back into the bladder by massaging the perineum; this simple method of preventing post-micturition dribble will save the man much discomfort and embarrassment as well as the expense of dry-cleaning and his wife's disapproval. Pelvic floor exercises should be taught to these men as it is their external sphincter mechanism which has become incompetent following transurethral surgery.

Toilet training may need to be discussed with the patient. Patterns of micturition depend on many factors. These may be medical (cardiac or renal failure), social (always go before you leave home) or psychological (it's my nerves, doctor). Lack of mobility will also influence the pattern, and the fear of pain involved in rising from a chair may well delay the act until it is too late. Similarly, those who have problems of urgency and urge incontinence due to an unstable bladder do not always anticipate the need to void. It is important that they understand their disability so that, if necessary, they may make more planned visits to the lavatory. Some men and women find the most difficult time to control their leakage is when rising from bed or from a chair. If pelvic floor exercises have been properly understood this is the time (on rising) to contract these muscles and stand up with confidence. Frequency of voiding is associated with a small capacity bladder. By increasing the fluid intake and delaying micturition under supervision the bladder will relax and accept a greater volume of urine. These measures are implemented in bladder drill (described later) for patients with unstable or hypersensitive bladders.

Many old people complain of nocturia. One episode during each night must be accepted as normal, but lack of sleep can seriously affect one's approach to the following day and, if there is an accumulation of broken nights, then a certain amount of despondence may set in. Nocturia can be a manifestation of a poor sleeper or the result of untreated cardiac failure. In most cases there are appropriate measures which may be taken to alleviate this symptom.

The amount of fluid which the patient drinks during the day needs careful assessment. Many people who have had pyelonephritis as children, an acute urinary infection or a period during which an indwelling catheter has been necessary will have been advised to drink copiously. Some continue to have a very high intake for many years after the event; others remember this advice when urinary symptoms recur. On checking a frequency/volume chart (see Chapter 2), it is often observed that the patient is drinking in excess of six pints (18 cups) daily in the belief that they are 'flushing their kidneys'. No wonder they complain of frequency of micturition!

A sensible fluid regime is therefore important. Tea or coffee may be found to have a particularly diuretic effect, in which case a bland alternative should be advised. If nocturia is a big problem then the withdrawal of fluid after 6.00 p.m. decreases this symptom. Certainly the need to void and the necessity for the bladder to be empty before going to bed must be stressed. Sleeplessness giving rise to nocturia can be helped by a light sedative which will break this habit.

Bed-wetting or nocturnal enuresis which has been found to occur at the same time each night is helped by an alarm clock set to ring prior to the act. In the young, an enuretic alarm may be used to good effect provided it is the child and not the family who wakes up to hear the bell ringing and change the sheets in the middle of the night. Again, these patients often have a small bladder capacity and this may be increased by a plentiful fluid intake.

Assessment is the key to successful management. The nurse must use this information to help her decide how best to help her patient. The emphasis is on the patient to take an active part in achieving continence. Already many of them will have been depressed by the doctor's pessimistic approach, and an attitude of optimism must be promoted at this stage.

Inpatient Assessment

In some patients assessment in a clinic is not adequate. The size of the problem may not become apparent to the nurse. This can be because of a muddled history or because certain aspects of the details obtained do not agree with the observations which are made. In other patients, it is not possible to establish a regime as an outpatient. It is for these people that a short stay in hospital is important. Here, as at the outpatient clinic, a pro forma has been found most useful; this gives continuity for the nursing staff, records are easier to keep and facts are more easily available for recall. It has been found that a five-day admission to hospital gives time to monitor the patients, to demonstrate different aids and to study the ability of the patient to manage these aids. A longer stay may seriously impede the elderly person's ability to return to an independent existence in the community.

Ideally, there should be beds allocated for urinary incontinence assessment in a general ward. Each patient has a junior nurse assigned to her. Rapport must be achieved early so that problems can be discussed easily. Routine investigations on admission include a flow rate, catheter specimen of urine and estimation of residual urine, and recordings are made of blood pressure, body weight and bowel habits.

Bladder Training. Frequency/volume charts will help to pinpoint habits of micturition and the patient must be encouraged to keep these herself. Also, the episodes of wetness should be indicated clearly. If nocturnal enuresis is a problem it may be necessary to check the bed half-hourly throughout the first couple of nights to ascertain at what time the incident occurs. From this chart, a pattern will emerge and bladder drill or toilet training can be established. The patient is reminded to void regularly at intervals which will anticipate the episodes of wetness. The intervals are increased as bladder control is gained. By appointing one nurse to take care of each patient the needs of the individual are maintained and regular four-hourly bedpan rounds become a pointless formality.

Drinking habits should be observed. Some may drink too much, others too little. If drug therapy is really needed (diuretics in particular) it must be noted so that these are taken at optimum times. Many elderly people have accumulated an amazing assortment of drugs over the years. This is an ideal time for medical assessment of the continuing need for therapy. Bowel habits must be studied — is there enough roughage in the diet or should simple laxatives be advised? Suppositories, an enema or manual removal of faeces may be needed to initiate a regular motion and thus alleviate severe urinary tract symptoms. The lethargy associated with chronic constipation may in itself lead to incontinence.

During the patient's stay in hospital the physiotherapist can make a most important contribution (see Appendix to Chapter 10). By assessing pelvic floor function and teaching both men and women the various methods by which control can be improved, a positive attempt may be made to restore continence. The small number of people involved lends itself to group therapy similar to the classes held in the post-natal ward.

If equipment is required this must be given while the patient is still under observation so that she may learn to manage it correctly herself. If the aid is found to be unsuitable then there is time during the five-day stay to try different devices or to make adaptations.

The patient should end her stay in hospital feeling optimistic about her ability to manage her incontinence on her own or with the help of her family. In some, management may be made easier by ensuring that they have the most suitable garments for their condition. Others will be continent after mastering the art of pelvic floor control.

Life-long nocturnal enuresis may be cured by a short admission to hospital, while other patients will be helped by ascertaining the usual hour of the episode and setting an alarm clock. Some patients will realise that they have lived with the fear of the disgrace associated with repeated incontinence after one isolated incidence. Some, for whom unnecessary precautions such as wearing protective garments have created an unjustified sense of security will need to regain regular voiding habits. Once their confidence is restored, protective clothing is no longer required. All those who are admitted will benefit by the knowledge that their problem is understood and shared by sympathetic and helpful nursing personnel. Their hospital admission may also be a most welcome break for those who shoulder the burden at home.

Home Assessment

Since the aim of management must be to enable the patient to remain in her own environment, a home visit by the nurse adviser, together with the community nurse, will give the greatest insight into the size of the problem. This visit provides continuity for the patient as well as invaluable instruction and encouragement to the community nurse.

Again, first impressions are important. Is there an overpowering smell of urine, are all the chairs covered with newspaper or are clothes badly stained? There may be the minimum of facilities. Some elderly people still have a bucket by the bed or in the living room as the only alternative to the lavatory down two flights of stairs or at the end of the garden. A moment of thought will show that provision of a commode or grab-bars fitted near the lavatory may be of greatest help. Mothers with enuretic children have been driven to distraction by having to hand-wash sheets and dry them in the living-room. The cost of a washing machine and tumble drier, which can be provided by the social services, pales into insignificance when compared to the disintegration of the family and the expense of hospital care which may be the alternative (see Chapter 13).

Are the chairs deep-seated and low, making easy access impossible or has the patient an old feather bed into which she has tumbled for the past 30 years and is now incapable of leaving till her daughter comes in the morning? Incontinence can have a devastating effect on domestic life. She may refuse to venture forth to do shopping or see friends. In becoming a recluse further problems arise. The offensive nature of the condition can be the culminating factor in the final breakdown of family support.

It is only by assessing the patients in their own setting that the whole problem is seen in context. Then the most appropriate methods of management may be found and continuing surveillance by the community nurse will help to improve the quality of life. Such a personalised service may appear to be an uneconomical way of approaching the problem, but apart from the nurse continence adviser, the personnel are already in post. *It is only expert guidance which is needed. Nothing is more costly than long-term hospital care and, for the patient, admission for incontinence is often the final straw.*

Aids to the Management of Incontinence

Many of the aids described in this section are listed, together with the names of suppliers, in Appendix C.

Pants and Pads

Although there is no perfect aid to offer the incontinent person, at least thorough assessment will mean that a logical choice can be made. No longer is he or she given what is available on the shelf but individual needs are catered for as nearly as possible. At present there is little which we can offer to a woman in the way of an incontinence device. Those that have been tried are not well tolerated. Pants and pads are the mainstay for the incontinent female to be used either permanently or during the period of retraining the bladder. Fortunately, the range of these garments is widening as the manufacturers receive more information on the acceptability and efficiency of their products when used under varying conditions. This is the only way in which improvements can be made. The more progressive manufacturers are grateful for the feedback which the patient can provide as a consumer.

A pilot study has shown that a variety of types of pants and pads are required so that individual needs may be met. Each type of pant has been developed with a particular need in mind and there are many considerations to be taken into account. The elderly are accustomed to wearing a different style from the young. Many men are reluctant to use garments designed principally for women. For those with urgency and urge incontinence the first priority is that both pants and pads may be removed with the utmost haste. The younger woman with stress incontinence is happiest with a feminine design which will hold a light pad capable of absorbing small quantities of urine but which will pass unnoticed under a tennis dress. A spina bifida child with total incontinence will need a pad capable of absorbing large quantities, particularly at night, and the pants will need to be as waterproof as possible and easy to put on. Some patients will rely on the security afforded by the protective clothing and they will be reluctant to respond to the normal desire to void. For these, increasing periods without pads in their own home may hasten the return to continence.

There are many considerations in assessing the suitability of the pants to the patient's requirements. The marsupial pants (Kanga; listed as 1. in Appendix C) with a waterproof pouch to hold the pad in position revolutionised incontinence wear. They are produced in designs for both young and old and there is a large range of sizes. A side opening is available if required and there are pants with Y-fronts for men. However, there are certain contra-indications:

(1) poor dexterity — two hands are required to place pad in pouch;
(2) heavy vaginal or urethral discharge, e.g. carcinoma of the pelvic organs;
(3) faecal incontinence;
(4) poor hygiene — not capable of washing garment;
(5) poor motivation — no incentive to change pad regularly because wetness cannot be appreciated.

The lightweight Helanca stretch pants (Molnlycke 2.) give adequate support to keep the recommended waterproof pad in place. There is a choice of three pads and the pants are also in three sizes, for light, medium and heavy loss, wash easily and are relatively low in cost. Their one contra-indication is the difficulty in pulling them on and off.

Plastic pants fill a definite need, particularly for patients who have a marked degree of incontinence. They are available in many sizes with elastic waistband and with a side opening to facilitate dressing. Contra-indications include:

(1) soreness and skin rashes;
(2) sweating;
(3) difficult to launder;
(4) tear easily.

Pads need to be selected by their capacity for absorbing urine and for their size. A large costly plastic-backed pad is not necessary where a sanitary towel will give adequate protection. When applying the special pad the outer edges should be folded upwards to create a gully which will receive the urine and prevent spillage before absorption occurs. The pad is the expensive part of the combination — a balance must be reached between changing it too often or so infrequently that the patient's skin is sore and chafed. Both day and night pads are available, the latter are larger and capable of absorbing larger volumes of urine.

Having decided that pants and pads will be used to keep the patient dry and comfortable either on a permanent basis or while more active methods are being considered, the correct size must be provided and a sufficient supply allocated. The patient and her family should understand the care of the garments, how the pad is fitted and the best method of laundering and pad disposal. They must know where to obtain further supplies, whether from the health centre, by post from manufacturers or over the counter from the chemist. A useful adjunct to meet these needs is a co-operation card carried at all times by the wearer. All details should be filled in by the clinic so that both hospital and community can provide the correct items (see p. 178). Financial considerations must be remembered. The cost of the pants, however expensive, is relatively small when compared with the number of pads which are required.

Appliances

Because of anatomical differences, appliances are a far more satisfactory method of management in men than in women. The few aids which have been produced for the female have resulted from many ingenious ideas, but none have been developed sufficiently to suit any but a very few women.

The decision to provide a male patient with an appliance will depend on his ability and willingness to manage the aid. Some will have to rely on the co-operation of their family and this, too, must be considered. Anatomically he may not be suited to a device. Gross obesity, a retracted penis or bilateral scrotal herniae will make the fitting difficult or impossible. There may be social factors which prevent this from being the management of choice.

There are many types of appliances available and the correct selection will depend on the patient. A comprehensive aid is the pubic pressure urinal (3.). This needs to be fitted by an expert and has various sizes of flanges and sheath diameters, different cones for ambulant and non-ambulant patients, extension tubing for wheelchair patients and a choice of rubber or webbing belts and plastic collecting bags. It is suitable for all types of incontinence, but, because of the relatively small size of the components it is not recommended for patients with poor eyesight or lack of dexterity or for those who are mentally confused.

A simpler device has the penile cone incorporated in a modified jock-strap (4.). This more closely resembles an article of clothing and is easier for the elderly or confused patient to manage.

A sheath or condom urinal (5.) is a very simple aid and is often the best method of management for the young paraplegic, for those confined to bed or in cases of temporary incontinence. Several sizes are available and attachment to the penis is by a strap (6.), strips of adhesive material (7.), or by special adhesive applied directly to the skin (8.).

Shaving of the pubic hair facilitates application and enhances the adhesive properties of the fixative. It is a lightweight device which is quick to apply and easy to manage provided that manual dexterity is good and that the attachment is not jeopardised by too much activity. For some, the use of a tubular bandage applicator will greatly facilitate correct positioning. Paul's tubing may also be used in some circumstances.

Many paraplegic centres have developed their own modifications. A simple sheath or condom can be attached to a piece of rubber tubing by a waterproof joint, and the rubber tubing then led to a collecting bag. The adaptation can be made to suit the individual with the correct length of connective tubing and has been found to be most useful.

Careful fitting of the appliance is as critical as the choosing of it, and must be done by an expert. The diameter and length of the penis and hip circumference need to be measured. Both the belt and understraps must be secured firmly but not too tightly so that the flange is held comfortably against the pubis. The cone top is selected according to the length of penis and type of use, a curved top for those who are ambulant and a straight top for sedentary patients.

If the urinal is to be used in bed the patient should be warned that a downward gradient must be maintained. This may necessitate raising the head of the bed or suggesting that the patient sleeps supported by many pillows. An alternative method of protection may be more convenient at night and it can be suggested that pants and pads or an incontinence sheet are substituted. An ill-fitting urinal will cause air to collect in the cone and collecting bag, a source of embarrassment and discomfort.

The need for careful training in the use of the appliance is even greater than for that given when supplying pants and pads. Directions are not always provided with the aid. Penile oedema will occur if the fitting is too tight and if the appliance is worn for too long during the early stages. Thus, men are advised to accustom themselves gradually — two hours on the first occasion is quite sufficient. An allergy to the latex rubber of the cone or the straps can cause skin rashes and soreness. In both cases the device must be removed until recovery is complete. Bathing the area with a dilute solution of Drapolene or using nongreasy barrier creams will alleviate these symptoms.

Although it may happen at any age youngsters, in particular, should be warned of the possibility of uncontrollable erections when first wearing an appliance. This can be particularly troublesome at night and may give rise to temporary penile congestion.

Good hygiene is essential. The pressure urinal needs to be emptied and rinsed thoroughly under cold running water. It is then advisable to soak the appliance in a weak solution of some disinfectant such as Milton before drying well and re-applying. Personal hygiene is equally important. Regular washing of the genitalia with thorough drying and, if required, a light application of zinc oxide talcum powder is advisable as well as shaving the pubic hair when using any type of urinal.

Included in the patient's education must be information on the different methods of attaching the appliance and the collecting bag. Straps are usually used and these may be fixed by buttons or by velcro. Cotton wool or gamgee may be used if extra padding is necessary. At night a larger collecting bag should be attached to allow for the extra volume of urine excreted during the sleeping hours.

The financial implications and the availability of supplies must be discussed. Until the patient is familiar with the device and has been satisfied that it works a single one will suffice. After the initial fitting it is advisable to see the patient again in two weeks. The patient must be told whom to contact in case of an emergency. Once the urinal has proved satisfactory a second one is supplied, but it is wise to re-assess before providing any further supplies. These may be obtained through the hospital, on prescription, or over the counter in a few shops. The patient should be warned of the hazards and disappointments likely from answering advertisements for the perfect appliance as seen in the 'small ads' of newspapers.

Although satisfactory management can be achieved in many men by using an appliance this method is never a substitute for active control, which should always be attempted in the first instance. For minor degrees of incontinence a simple dribble bag or disposable pouch may be used. This is intended for very slight nocturnal enuresis or post-micturition dribble.

Long-term Catheterisation

In both men and women with severe urinary incontinence it may be necessary to consider long-term catheterisation as the most effective method of management. The decision to use this method must be made by the doctor in charge of the patient. Whether the catheter is passed by the doctor or nurse (either male or female) depends on availability, policy, training and to some extent the patient's preference. Many nurses both in the community and in hospital are considerably more experienced in passing urethral catheters than the majority of junior hospital doctors or some family doctors. In order to have an overall standard of expertise it has been our practice to hold practical sessions for nurses and to issue a certificate of competence. This will indicate the willingness of male and female nurses to catheterise both men and women.

The decision having been made, the practicalities must be considered. The variety of catheters on the market suggests that the perfect one has yet to be produced. Also, it is indicative of the amount of money which is involved. New catheters are constantly being produced and need careful and critical appraisal. Expense must always be a consideration. The catheters which are used in the long-term management of incontinence are self-retaining. They are made of plastic or latex with a latex rubber balloon, or of plastic with various additives such as Teflon, and more recently silicone has been used either to coat the catheter or as the sole material. These are relatively non-reactive and have a longer life. As in the other aids to incontinence, each has a specific use and none can be considered as a multi-purpose catheter. There are now many firms producing short catheters for women to use.

The catheters selected for the initial catheterisation should be inexpensive (e.g. latex coated). If it is well tolerated, and there is no leakage or blockage problem after the first two weeks, then is the time to replace it with a long-term silicone catheter. Prices range from under £1.00 for the latex catheter to between £3.50 and £8.00 for the silicone catheters. Careful consideration must be given to economic aspects as the patient may require a considerable number of catheter changes before the optimum method of management is found. In our experience the expensive silicone catheters have no advantage over the cheaper latex-coated products.

The size of the catheter as well as the amount of fluid used to fill the retaining balloon are important considerations in catheter management. By tradition catheter circumference has been measured by the French Gauge (FG) or Charrière. A committee from the British Standards Institute is currently meeting to standardise the measurement and to introduce metrication. We have found that either 14 FG or 18 FG are the only two sizes required for routine long-term catheter drainage.

The volume of fluid used to fill the retaining balloon is another controversial point. The amount written on the catheter (e.g. 5 ml, 10 ml, 30 ml) is the maximum balloon capacity as quoted by the manufacturers. It is not an indication of the volume necessary to retain the catheter. Many bladders which have been drained continuously are only capable of slight distension. If 30 ml is its maximum capacity, the bladder will then contract to try to extrude the catheter. Detrusor instability will cause painful abdominal cramp and leakage around the balloon. At this stage, a decrease in the amount of fluid in the balloon, rather than an increase, is more likely to keep the patient dry. Five ml to ten ml of fluid in the balloon is usually sufficient to retain the catheter. Nurses have created havoc by increasing catheter size and balloon volume in a useless attempt to produce leakage-proof catheter drainage. Indeed, if the patient is known to have an unstable bladder, as in those with multiple sclerosis, a certain amount of leakage may have to be accepted. In some of these patients an exacerbation may be expected after changing the catheter. Bladder relaxants such as emepronium bromide, flavoxate hydrochloride or orciprenaline, may reduce detrusor activity and thus decrease the amount of incontinence. They are worth a trial in difficult cases.

Satisfactory catheter management is dependent on the patient or his family understanding the basic principles which are involved. It is elementary domestic plumbing and the majority of people understand that water does not run uphill, that a kink or a twist in the tube will create a blockage, that milking a tube will clear a temporary blockage and, that if a circuit is broken, an air-lock is likely to occur. These facts must be explained as well as the relationship of the catheter to day-to-day functions. There is nothing to prevent the patient having a bath, provided that the collecting bag is disconnected and replaced by a spigot. When the patient sits or alters his position the tube must be watched for twisting or accidental detachment by body pressure or locking between the knees. Intercourse is usually possible for women, but for sexually active men this can be difficult. It may be better to teach the man or his partner to do intermittent catheterisation; alternatively a supra-pubic catheter may be more acceptable. A regular fluid intake and regular bowel movement must be encouraged for all catheter users.

The frequency with which a catheter will need changing varies with the reason for its introduction and with the type which is used. It is recommended that the latex-coated catheter is changed at two- to three-week intervals although in practice this can be extended to at least eight weeks. The long-term silicone catheters appear to drain satisfactorily for up to three months in the majority of people. There is no doubt that irrespective of the type of catheter or its management some patients are recurrent 'blockers'. In any large series there will be a group whose catheters become encrusted irrespective of management. These are probably the ones for whom bladder washouts should be considered. Tap water is readily available and, if guaranteed fit for drinking, is clean and very suitable for this purpose. The intelligent patient or his family are soon able to perform washouts if the community nurse is unable to attend.

It must be accepted that most people with a long-term indwelling catheter will develop a chronic urinary infection. This is usually localised to the bladder and the organisms most commonly cultured are *E. Coli* or a mixture of indigenous flora. Provided there is no evidence of systemic infection the existing bacteriuria does not need treatment (see p. 40).

Success with catheter management is as dependent on a satisfactory collecting bag as it is on the catheter. Variations in their manufacture are legion, each having been developed for a specific purpose. The essential is to have a bag which holds sufficient urine, is simple to attach to the catheter and is held in a position which suits the individual and can be emptied readily. The complications arise when a different type of bag is provided and its eccentricities have not been explained. The inlet may look identical to the outlet. The outlet may be closed by a screw, a tap, a spigot or a number of different methods. These can all be managed by the users if they are accustomed to them but a change can mean blockage, stoppage and alarm where there is lack of dexterity, mental aptitude or failing eyesight.

Each patient should be provided with a day bag and a night bag. The day bag has a capacity of up to 500 ml. It must be provided with a suitable method of attachment to the patient. Many men prefer a long connecting tube so that the collecting bag can be worn below a baggy pair of trousers. For women this is not acceptable. Some will wear the bag on the inner aspect of the thigh below long, loose skirts, but women's thighs are notoriously ill-shaped for attachment, being conical with the apex downwards. For some a waist belt with attachments similar to the old-fashioned suspender belt or a modified knicker with a pouch makes a more suitable alternative. Once again a co-operation card containing all the details will prove invaluable as a link between hospital and community. It will prevent many unnecessary emergency visits to hospital. It is possible to find a satisfactory and discreet method of collecting urine across the floor. Personal dignity must be respected.

The collecting bags are disposable, but should be used until they look as if they need renewing (one to two weeks). They should be washed nightly in soapy water and rinsed well before replacing. The night bag has a larger capacity (500 ml or more). It can be attached to a night stand, special modifications being available for divan beds. There are many different types of straps for attachment and here it must be by trial and error that the individual requirements are met.

Arrangements for the continued care of the patient must be clearly defined. It may be the responsibility of the community nurse to change the catheter at home or there may be a catheter clinic in the local hospital. The patient must know whom to call in case of emergencies and the trained staff involved must know which size and type of catheter is most satisfactory for the individual. Ideally, all patients should have a sterile pack and spare catheter available at home. A small book on the catheter and its management with a page for personal information should be provided for each user. If incontinence is the reason for catheter management there should be no need for emergency visits to hospital should the catheter become blocked. All that is necessary is for the catheter to be removed. Leakage can usually be tolerated until help is available. In some cases the patient or his family will be able to deflate the balloon provided they have been taught correctly. Certainly the community nurse on call or the family doctor will be able to manage this crisis. Subsequently, a routine appointment can be made for the patient to attend for re-catheterisation during clinic hours.

Supra-pubic Catheterisation

Supra-pubic catheter drainage is now an accepted method of short-term management following surgery. In certain situations it has an application in the long-term management of incontinence. In those women with severe neurological disablement as in advanced multiple sclerosis this is a technique which has been used with satisfactory results. The catheter is passed supra-pubically using a stab incision under cystoscopic control with the patient under general anaesthesia. As yet there are no catheters adapted for this method and an ordinary Foley catheter FG 18 is used with 10 ml in the retaining balloon. Once a fistula has been established the catheter may be changed routinely by an experienced nurse.

The method has many advantages — it is simple, reversible, convenient and relatively successful in the cases of which we have experience. Disadvantages include the risk of infection, leakage around the catheter and *per urethram* and blockage. If the catheter falls out during the early days or is left out for any length of time it will be difficult to replace. Closure of the urethra will stop troublesome leakage but will make

Figure 9.1: Co-operation Card   Front

Rear

CATHETER CHANGES:—

Date	Cath. size	Comment

CO-OPERATION CARD FOR INDWELLING CATHETER

Always keep this card available.

Always bring it with you when visiting your doctor, the hospital, or when requesting supplies.

NAME

ADDRESS

G.P.

It is important to keep a new spare catheter and several bags at home. Most catheters are now obtainable on prescription from your G.P.

M.1109 A

Inside

CONSULTANT

HOSPITAL

UNIT NUMBER

TYPE OF CATHETER

SIZE

BALLOON VOLUME

TYPE OF BAG _____ CAPACITY

SOURCE OF SUPPLY

Medical Indication

To be filled in by Nurse:—

DAILY URINE OUTPUT

IS CONSTIPATION A PROBLEM?

IS BLADDER IRRIGATION REQUIRED? Yes/No

IF SO, TECHNIQUE:—

IN EMERGENCY, CONTACT:—

Your General Practitioner/Community Nurse or Urology Clinic

_____ Hospital

Telephone No. _____ Exn

urethral catheterisation impossible as an emergency procedure.

This is a technique of management which needs more time for proper evaluation, but should certainly be considered before subjecting the patient to major surgery and the finality of an ileal conduit.

Clean Intermittent Self-catheterisation

This is a method used to manage the patient with incontinence due to overflow or with a reflex bladder. History has turned full circle since the days when men kept their own silver catheters in their top hats and circumnavigated the urethral strictures caused by the gonococcus in order to relieve themselves. Now intermittent self-catheterisation is used extensively by males and females with spina bifida and by paraplegics. It has proved to be an effective alternative in women with multiple sclerosis who maintain their manual dexterity and in women with large hypotonic bladders who fail to void to completion and who subsequently complain of frequency and incontinence.

Sufficient patient or family motivation is essential and each will find their own most convenient method for passing the catheter. Some find a mirror is useful. More often it is done by feeling for the urethral meatus with the patient sitting on the lavatory seat, in the bath, or on the side of the bed. Until the technique has been perfected it is advisable to use a sterile disposable short catheter and a pair of sterile disposable gloves at each attempt. Subsequently, the same catheter may be re-used after washing in cold water and being placed in a suitable container. The number of times that this procedure needs to be undertaken varies from once a week to two hourly and is dependent on the patient's age and the type of bladder dysfunction. For children with spina bifida it is recommended that once over the age of two years the parent and subsequently the child empties the bladder at two-hourly intervals.

Occlusive Devices

There are various occlusive devices for men, all of which are modifications of the penile clamp. They are mentioned only to be discounted. None is satisfactory except as a very short-term method of management. Penile necrosis and fistula formation are the recognised complications.

Women have been accustomed to wearing ring pessaries for the control of vaginal prolapse for many years. Their effectiveness when used to prevent urinary incontinence is doubtful. However, some women who have a minor degree of stress incontinence find that a tampon-shaped pessary made of foam rubber by Rocket Ltd (15.) will help both to absorb small quantities of urine and to support the posterior urethra. Similarly, some have found that an ordinary tampon is enough to prevent leakage.

Probably the best occlusive device available for women is the Eschmann or Bonnar (17.) inflatable device. After insertion into the vagina a balloon is inflated and elevates the bladder neck and proximal urethra. This is a well-designed and nicely presented piece of equipment. For well-motivated women with a good degree of manual dexterity it can be a successful method of maintaining continence during physical exercise. It is, however, difficult to deflate quickly at times of extreme urgency and many elderly people find it impossible to insert or to retain in position.

The electrical stimulation devices have been mentioned in Chapter 2. Recent trials have suggested that both stress and urge incontinence can be treated logically with different frequencies. Their success rate has been limited by technical problems and lack of patient motivation. Certainly they are not indicated as a method of management in the elderly incontinent person.

Receptacles

Besides the appliances which have already been described there are various urinals and commodes specifically manufactured to facilitate the collection of urine and therefore help to maintain continence. Because of basic anatomical differences these are more easily designed for men than women. Most male urinals consist of a flattened bottle and some designs have a non-return valve at the neck to prevent spillage (18.). There are some excellent products which are watertight, discreet and disposable (19.) — very useful for long coach journeys when facilities are limited and where appropriate occasions for relief only occur at long intervals.

Considerable research has been involved in designing appropriate collecting devices for women. The St Peter's Boat (20.) is an egg-shaped dish with a handle which may be slipped easily between the legs. The Suba-Seal (21.) is another female urinal which has a handle and is designed to be non-spill. A more recent addition is the Feminal (22.), produced as a 'handbag' urinal. This has a plastic frame contoured to fit the female anatomy to which is attached a disposable plastic bag for urine collection. In theory, it should be possible to use it when standing, sitting or lying. In practice this can be difficult because of obesity, lack of mobility and lack of dexterity. However, it is certainly the most useful device of its kind being marketed.

A special piece of equipment has been designed for those who have difficulty in directing the flow of urine. This is a simple cone, open at both ends and shaped appropriately at the wider end so that it may be pressed against the perineum in either men or women. It has been found most useful in those women with severe vaginitis or a scarred perineal area following radical vulvectomy. Also, those men who have bilateral scrotal herniae or who have a retracted penis are able to direct the flow of urine and prevent dribbling during voiding.

The commode, once a common piece of furniture in the hospital and in the home, became a rarity as plumbing has improved. Its presence in the ward was thought to be offensive and unhygienic when nursing routine was strictly clinical. Yet, there has never been an adequate number of lavatories provided in hospitals, particularly for the elderly. There was a time when mobilisation of the patient was considered of such paramount importance that old people where expected to walk the length of an old-fashioned ward when seized by the desire to void. No wonder that there were many disasters on the way. Old people with unstable bladders, walking with the aid of sticks or helped by a well-meaning physiotherapist, cannot be expected to inhibit detrusor contractions as well as concentrate on ambulation.

There are a large number of commodes on the market and most are acceptable as pieces of furniture. Some are available from the voluntary services as well as the health service. Their presence both in the home and in the ward is a necessity for those who have urge incontinence and are unable to reach the lavatory because of lack of mobility (see Appendix C).

Bed Protection

For those who are bed-bound or chair-bound it is often necessary to protect the bedding or the furniture. Although plastic sheeting is often useful it is not comfortable, is not absorbent and it has a most deleterious effect on the patient's skin. There are many incontinence sheets made of absorbent materials such as paper, blocked wood-pulp or cellulose with a waterproof backing which can be placed next to the patient's skin. These vary in their absorbency but there is none that keeps the patient completely dry and surveys have reported that there is only a 40 per cent success rate in keeping the bedding dry.

The Kylie sheet (23.) has been developed using a hydrophobic material which separates the patient from the absorbent pad, thus helping to keep the skin dry. These wash well and go some way to fulfil a need for those with nocturnal incontinence.

One of the most socially unacceptable aspects of urinary incontinence is that of the associated smell. This is the reason for the majority of sufferers becoming ostracised by society. Yet there are various most effective neutralising deodorants which are available. Nilodor (24.) is perhaps the most satisfactory of these products. Advice on this particular aspect is a vital part of counselling on the management of urinary incontinence for the patient, the relatives and those in charge of old people's homes.

A full list of those items mentioned in this chapter is given in Appendix C.

Note

1. Editor's note: since the publication of the first edition of this book there are many more nurses in Britain already filling this role, some attached to specialised units and others working in various other capacities in the health service. It is hoped that eventually there will be an advisory nurse of this kind in each health district. See also: Isaacs, B. (1979), 'The Management of Urinary Incontinence in Departments of Geriatric Medicine', *Health Trends, 11*, 42-4.

10 RE-EDUCATION OF THE MUSCLES OF THE PELVIC FLOOR

Angela M. Shepherd

Re-education of the muscles of the pelvic floor is one of the simplest and most rewarding methods of regaining bladder control for those with troublesome but not severe urinary incontinence. Over the years it has been established by physiotherapists as a useful adjunct to recovery in mothers during the puerperal period. In 1951 Kegel suggested that good results could also be obtained when this treatment was given to debilitated elderly women.[1] It is a technique which has fallen behind as a method of management, perhaps because of poor patient selection or because of lack of teaching motivation. Few recent controlled trials have been reported from which we can judge its efficacy.

As has been stated in Chapter 1, the components for the primary control of continence are the peri-urethral meatus and the external urethral sphincter mechanism. There is no distinct circular band of muscle fibres as there is in the anal sphincter. The nervous control is mostly by parasympathetic nerves with very few, if any, striated muscle fibres capable of voluntary contraction. The pelvic floor muscles (levator-ani and transverse-perinei) control the ability to stop voiding in mid-stream. It is probable that a constant state of tension existing in these muscles also helps to maintain the resting but active state of continence. Electromyographic studies have shown that, except during voiding, there is always some electrical activity present in the peri-urethral musculature. It is a fact that men, using basically the same muscle group, have no difficulty in directing their stream or stopping completely if required. Those who have to supervise the collection of mid-stream specimens of urine will know that in many women this is a wet and messy operation. By contracting the muscles of the pelvic floor men are able to double the resting urethral pressure, yet many European women, whether dry or wet, have the greatest difficulty in controlling their stream and few can raise the resting urethral pressure by more than 20 per cent.

There would appear to be a basic geographic difference in the incidence of stress incontinence among women. Whether this is racial or cultural or due to different standards of hygiene is not obvious. Certainly this type of urinary leakage is unusual among the Bantu of southern Africa, but it is also a rare complaint among the more fasti-dious Malay and Chinese people. Perhaps the following facts provide an explanation. Lavatory seats are a rarity among the rural people and they squat to void. Hence they need to control their stream and if they mis-aim they have to stop and start again. Secondly, although not a universal characteristic, many others teach their daughters pelvic floor control for use in sexual stimulation. A vaginal assessment will demon-strate a good contraction of the muscles in many, an ability which is rarely found among Western women. Only 43 per cent of those attend-ing a gynaecological clinic in the United Kingdom were able to contract their perineal muscles on command, irrespective of whether their symptoms were of genital or urological origin.

Genuine stress incontinence (leakage on coughing, laughing, or hitting a ball) is the most common type of leakage among women. It can also occur in men, when it may follow prostatic surgery. Elec-trical stimulation of the perineal muscles followed by exercise has been advocated for years as a treatment for this type of urinary leakage. The results depend entirely on the motivation of both the patient and the instructor. Various types of electrical impulse can be used – the aim being to produce the maximum muscle contraction for the minimum sensory discomfort. The older faradic battery has been replaced by interrupted direct current with variable pulse duration and speed and interferential current is being used in a few centres where good results have been reported. However, in more recent trials the use of this type of current alone or together with exercises has not added any improvement to the results.[2]

The rationale behind electrical stimulation being included in the regime of re-education of the pelvic floor is that it increases the blood supply, it can break down any adhesions which may follow surgery, it increases the resting tone of the muscles and perhaps most important of all it restores cortical awareness. Thus, the patient is able to feel the contraction of the pelvic floor by electrical stimulation and is able to repeat this voluntarily.

The levator-ani muscles, under voluntary control, possess the ability to stop voiding in mid-stream. They are classified as having 'quick-twitch' muscle fibres capable of responding rapidly, and fatiguing quickly. Re-education of this group may be achieved by active exercise alone. The peri-urethral muscles maintain the resting urethral tone, and like the other postural muscles of the body this group is of the 'slow twitch' type. They are capable of sustained contraction and do not fatigue easily. Physiologists suggest that these two different types of muscle fibres possess the ability to convert from one to the other if their basic function is altered. Hence, it is logical to assume that resting urethral tone may be increased by improving the function of the pelvic floor muscles.

The first priority is to be sure that the patient not only understands the reason for re-education of the pelvic floor muscles but is also sufficiently aware of her perineum to produce a voluntary contraction. There is only one way to be sure that the order has been interpreted correctly. If two fingers are placed just within the introitus the instructor will be able to assess the presence of a muscle contraction. There are many ways to encourage the patient to establish good muscle control, but the emphasis should be on creating an awareness of a constant pelvic floor contraction which is continuously maintained in the upright position and which is fortified at the first hint of a cough, sneeze or on hitting a tennis ball. It should be possible to re-establish this reflex by conditioning and repetition. After all, it is usually the parous woman who has problems. During the 40 weeks of pregnancy her perineal muscles will have relaxed and the pelvic supports will have stretched. A large non-compressible object (the baby's head) will have slowly forced its way through what was an intact pelvic floor. It is small wonder that whereas men are able to create high urethral pressures and have good control of their urinary flow when they contract their muscles, this ability is lost in many women.

A combination of electrical stimulation together with intensive re-education of the pelvic floor muscles is a highly successful method of regaining urinary control. In our recent study of 44 women, all of whom had proven incompetence of the bladder neck, 39 were so much improved that surgical treatment was unnecessary. Their ages ranged from 18 years to 73 years. Not only did their episodes of wetness become minimal but both day and night time frequency were appreciably reduced.

The strength of the pelvic muscles may be tested by a perineometer, as was described by Kegel (see Appendix to this chapter). Patients are most encouraged when they can compare initial readings with those obtained as the ability improves. However, the perfect measuring device has yet to be designed and digital assessment is the only alternative: providing the same person is gauging the improvement this too can be reliable. Efforts are still underway to produce a perineometer or pelvic exerciser which is robust, aesthetically acceptable and economic. Based on that of Kegel (see Appendix to this chapter) workers have had various ideas. Of the two illustrated each have their advantages and both have proved their worth in controlled trials (see Figures 10.1 and 10.2).

Figure 10.1: Prototype of Perineometer Developed by Craig Medical (not available commercially)

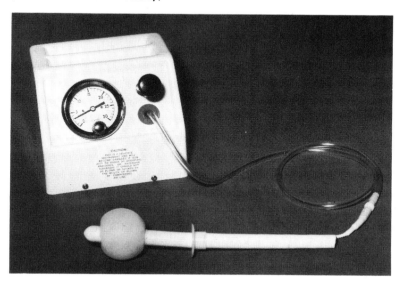

Figure 10.2: Prototype of Perineometer Developed by T. Floyd in Conjunction with the Clinical Investigation Unit, Ham Green Hospital, Bristol

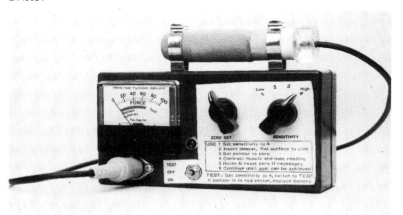

	Trial	Control
Dry	8	3
Improved	2	3
Same	1	5

These ideas have yet to be accepted by a manufacturer as a product which will be economic to produce. However, there has been worldwide interest and such a device should be available to every nurse, physiotherapist and doctor who is interested in conservative methods of management of stress incontinence.

Although it is more conventional to combine electrical stimulation with active re-education, there are those who advocate either one or the other. A detailed description of treatment by muscular re-education is given in the Appendix to this chapter. Successful results depend largely on the correct selection of patients with genuine stress incontinence who are well motivated. The other vital ingredient is a teacher, be it nurse, physiotherapist, doctor or non-medical enthusiast, who understands the rationale, believes in this method of treatment and is able to give time to explain to the patient what is expected of her.

Note

1. Kegel, A.H. (1951), 'Physiologic Therapy for Urinary Stress Incontinence', *J.A.M.A.*, *146*, 915-17.
2. Wilson, P.D., Al Samarral, T., Deakin, M., Kolbe, E. and Brown, A.D.G. (1984), 'The Value of Physiotherapy in Female Genuine Stress Incontinence', Proceedings, International Continence Society (Innsbruck), 156-8.

APPENDIX: A PROGRAMME FOR RE-EDUCATION

Dorothy Mandelstam

The importance of the functions of the pelvic floor has been referred to above and in other chapters. Treatment for stress incontinence can be by physiotherapeutic measures or surgery or both, but there is only one published trial of physiotherapy techniques (see Chapter 10).

Active muscular exercise on its own has proved effective, and has the added advantage of not requiring the patient's frequent attendance at a hospital. As in all treatments, a diagnosis and correct selection of patients is important.

Indications. Most women with stress incontinence exhibit poor tone and laxity of the pelvic floor musculature. In many there appears no gross anatomical abnormality and in the absence of severe fascial damage, as evidenced by a patulous shortened prolapsed urethra, non-operative treatment can be effective.

Aim. The aim is to strengthen the deep fascio-muscular layer of the pelvic floor, consisting of the levator-ani with particular attention to the pubo-coccygeal component. These muscles, while mainly supportive, can be used to augment sphincteric action. In addition, the other sphincteric muscles, the transverse perineal and the anal sphincter are made to contract, their action being concomitant.

Treatment

The patient is given a very complete but simple description of the pelvic floor and the aims of treatment, followed by a digital examination assessing the tone of the levator-ani, and also instruction in the use of the muscles. Once initiated, the patient is encouraged to contract muscles slowly four times. This is repeated hourly or at other convenient intervals and can be done without disturbance to daily routine. To assess progress a monthly check is all that is required and the average length of treatment is three months.

The Perineometer

The perineometer (see Figure A.1), which was devised by A.H. Kegel[1] was used as a visual teaching aid, especially for the patient with little muscle awareness. This is no longer available from the USA, but attempts are being made to produce one similar (see Chapter 10).

It consists of a compressible rubber air chamber, 8 cm long and 2 cm in diameter, connected by rubber tubing to a manometer. The chamber is stretched over a slender rigid tube with an air vent which connects it with the tubing. The base is fitted with a round shield which rests against the perineum so limiting its position in the vagina. As the appropriate muscles contract, the manometer registers any increase of air pressure within the chamber. This affords a visual guide so that the end results of correctly directed efforts can be assessed. It is also a means of recording progress.

Figure A.1: The Perineometer

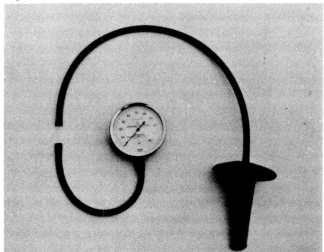

Instructions for Patients

If there is no specialist physiotherapist available, the following instructions can be given to patients to help them become aware of the pelvic muscles:[2]

(1) Tighten and release the muscles around the back passage.
(2) While passing urine, stop the flow and notice the sensation of muscle contraction in the front.
(3) Once both these movements are learnt, start by contracting the back passage and then the front part. The pelvic muscles work as a whole and are to be contracted slowly four times. Repeat this every hour or as often as possible. This can be carried out at any time, e.g. waiting for a bus, watching television etc.

After two or three weeks' practice, there will be an awareness of the sensation of closure of the passage (back and front) and the feeling of drawing up the pelvic floor in front. The abdominal, thigh and buttock muscles should not be tightened and legs should remain uncrossed, so that the pelvic muscles alone can be felt. It is a distinct and separate movement from the other muscles and can be checked (while in the bath) by placing one finger into the vagina and contracting the muscles. The exercise is to be continued daily for three months.

Selected Patients

Table A.1 shows illustrative examples of patients who responded to this treatment without surgery.

Table A.1: Illustrative Cases of Stress Incontinence Treated

Name	Age	Parity	Duration of Symptom	Clinical Findings	Operation	Other Factors
Mrs A	37	2	5 years	Cystocele Rectocele	nil	Obese
				Levator response absent		
Mrs S	57	2	Since childbirth	Cystocele	nil	Hypertension Normal micturating cystogram.
Mrs Ga	55	3	2 years	1 Prolapse	nil	—
Mrs Se	55	4	7 years	Cystocele	nil	—

Women in this table are all parous. If obesity exists weight loss is advocated. The second example (Mrs S) shows a patient who had stress for many years. The micturating cystogram was normal and the symptom was relieved. Other examples are typical of women benefiting from this treatment.

The second group (Table A.2) are women who had stress incontinence after surgery and in whom the symptom disappeared with muscular re-education.

Table A.2: Illustrative Cases Treated after Previous Surgery

Name	Age	Parity	Duration of symptom	Clinical findings	Operation	Other factors
Mrs M	70	2	7 years	Hypotonic levator muscle	Vag hyst	—
Mrs G	52	2	2 years	Levator awareness absent	Vag hyst	Obese, hypertensive, normal cystogram
Mrs F	43	3	Before surgery	Levator awareness poor	Ant post repair	—
Mrs C	67	4	Post-op	—	Vag hyst	Adequate control before surgery

In the first case (Mrs M) the symptom persisted after a vaginal hysterectomy. In the second, who was overweight and hypertensive, the symptom recurred after a vaginal hysterectomy. Urodynamic investigation revealed that when the urethral pressure profile measurements were repeated after muscle re-education the resting urethral pressure had more than doubled. The last case is an example of a patient who developed stress incontinence after surgery.

A Retrospective Survey, 1970-6 (Norfolk and Norwich Hospital)

Table A.3 shows results produced by Sheila M. Harrison, MCSP, of a group of 212 patients with stress incontinence treated by muscular re-education.

Table A.3: Patients with Stress Incontinence Treated by Muscle Re-education

	No.	%
1. Success	199	93
Failure	13	7
	212	
2. Causes of failure		
Severe cough	3	
Gross obesity	1	
Inappropriate selection in gynaecological clinic (too much utero-vaginal prolapse)	9	
	13	
3. Duration of successful treatments		
3-5 months	154	72
6-9 months	45	23
	199	
4. Pre- or post-menopausal		
Pre-menopausal	154	72
Post-menopausal	58	28
	212	
5. Previous failed repairs for stress incontinence (SI), then treated by muscular re-education (16 out of 212)		
One previous repair for SI	11	
Two previous repairs for SI	2	
Three previous repairs for SI	3	
	16*	
6. Obesity in group of 212		
Normal weight	133	59
5 kg overweight**	79	41
	212	

*all successful.
**standard tables height/weight.
Source: Reproduced with kind permission from Downie, P.A. (ed.), *Cash's Textbook of Physiotherapy in Some Surgical Conditions*, 6th edn (Faber and Faber, London and Boston, 1979).

A number of points of interest arise from these results:

(1) initial diagnosis of stress incontinence was made clinically —
cystometry was not used;

(2) in all but 16 cases (previous repairs) muscular re-education was
the first treatment of choice; and

(3) stress incontinence which persists through one or more operations can frequently be cured by muscular re-education of the
pelvic floor muscles.

Notes

1. Kegel, A.H. (1948), The Non-surgical Treatment of Genital Relaxation',
Annals West. Med. Surg., 2(5), 213-16.
2. For reading to recommend to patients, I suggest: Montgomery, E. (1974),
Regaining Bladder Control (Wright, Bristol).

11 REHABILITATIVE NURSING

Elizabeth C. Clay

Incontinence is a symptom requiring investigation, a correct diagnosis and properly-conducted treatment. Failure to provide adequate treatment results in the social rejection of the individuals concerned, who may find themselves segregated from home, family and friends (see Chapter 13). This isolation can usually be avoided or overcome by rehabilitative nursing management, which may be practised with suitable modifications with patients of any age.

The aim of rehabilitation is the resocialisation of the patient, either by alleviating the condition, or concealing it by successful protective management. In the Department of Geriatric Medicine of Birmingham's Dudley Road Hospital three nursing procedures relating to urinary incontinence have been devised and conducted by nurses with medical support. The choice of procedure depends on the individual needs of the patient.

These nursing procedures are practised when there is no other effective medical treatment. They may also be used in conjunction with treatment.

The nursing assessment of the patient not only identifies nursing problems but can provide accurate information contributing to the diagnosis. Other members of the multidisciplinary team are encouraged to participate in these nursing procedures when patients are in their departments for treatment. This ensures continuity of the regime which is vital to ultimate success.

A Basis for Rehabilitation

Nurses and other members of the multidisciplinary team must be free of those cultural and personal prejudices and those traditional hospital practices which obstruct rehabilitation (see Chapter 7, p. 113). Degradation of the patient's adult status is unacceptable. The need for empathy is never so great as in disabling conditions, which, in themselves alone, inhibit the patient's efforts and initiative to recover. A respectful and tolerant approach is basic to obtaining the patient's confidence and co-operation.

195

Patients should not be hurried, and the ward routine should be geared to the patient's rehabilitation requirements. Adherence to a rigid routine indicates that staff have not taken into account the individual needs of the patients.

The hospital environment should be homely rather than luxurious, adequately heated, ventilated and with normal comforts. There should be an adequate provision of lavatories spacious enough to enable patients to manoeuvre with walking aids or in wheelchairs, where necessary lavatory seats should be raised, and there should be wall-bars to facilitate patients' mobility. A commode, urine bottle or bedpan should be placed at the bedside at night. Accessibility of facilities reduces the anxiety which patients feel when they have to rely solely on attracting someone's attention.

The patient's personal appearance reflects self-respect. Hair and skin should be well cared for. Normal clothing should be worn. Women should wear suitable stockings or single-leg tights and their dresses should cover their knees when sitting. Easy removal of clothes by velcro fastening instead of a zip or buttons may make the difference between continence and incontinence when the call to void is urgent. Pants should always be worn. Patients should never be placed on a pad on a chair, for this advertises incontinence and affects self-respect and rehabilitation. Privacy should always be ensured.

As it is important that nurses find time to sit and talk to patients for reasonable periods, a change of attitude is required on the part of senior staff so that this is not regarded as time-wasting. There is no substitute for human companionship and five or ten minutes of the nurse's time will suffice. Anyone coming in contact with patients should give a friendly greeting. Neglect of these normal courtesies can reduce a patient to feeling less than human. Open visiting by relatives and friends is very important as it brings increased companionship.

The Nursing Team

Education and training, as well as a high degree of vocational dedication, are essential for this most difficult form of nursing. Rehabilitation depends upon the development of good relations between members of the multidisciplinary team, patients, their friends, and relatives. The nursing skills necessary for this rehabilitation include the ability to make accurate observations and recordings, and to interpret the results; and then to plan and implement the rehabilitative nursing procedures, and to evaluate and consult with all members of the multidisciplinary team in a mutually supportive action. The nursing team should work with therapeutic optimism, with full appreciation of the needs of the patient, using discretion, patience and encouragement during the periods of observation. Nurses inexperienced in rehabilitation require initiation into the psychological implications of incontinence. A denial by the patient of the existence of incontinence is common, and all kinds of excuses for wetness are offered. These rationalisations are, in fact, desperate attempts to preserve self-respect, and will emphasise to the nurse the importance of avoiding attitudes of condescension and reproach.

Assessment of the Patient

It will be apparent that any scheme of rehabilitation must be preceded by a general assessment of the patient, and a form (Figure 11.1) is a useful means of recording this on admission. It also serves to indicate rehabilitation needs. It is important to secure the co-operation of the patient by a careful and detailed explanation of the aims and procedures of the rehabilitation programme. Time taken over this is never wasted, as any impression of impatience can inhibit participation.

The Preliminary Check

This is based on two-hourly observation for the full 24 hours, to discover whether the patient is wet or dry, and this is then recorded on a chart (see Figure 11.2). The patient is then asked to pass urine, and the result also recorded. If toilet facilities are declined, this is also recorded. If at this two-hourly check the patient is found to be incontinent, the time can be shortened; if on the other hand toilet facilities are not needed so frequently, the interval can be lengthened. It is by these adjustments that a pattern of micturition will emerge. This may take anything from 3 to 14 days, and in some cases, longer.

On the basis of information recorded on the chart, patients with a defined pattern of micturition can now be considered for habit re-training. The aim of this is to produce a socially acceptable toilet rhythm by retraining the bladder, from the starting point of the pattern shown. The chart itself will be the tool for the job. Nursing staff will require full instruction in the use of the chart, and time to practise using it under supervision.

Figure 11.1: Nursing Assessment of the Patient on Admission

NURSING ASSESSMENT OF THE PATIENT ON ADMISSION

Diagnosis (Medical): _____

Identification of Nursing Problems: _____

Function	Tick where applicable.		REMARKS	Rehabilitation Date Begun.
	Normal	Abnormal		
COMMUNICATION: Interests				
Dislikes				
Activities				
Hearing				
Understanding				
Speech				
Sight				
AWARENESS: Place				
Time				
MOBILITY: Feeding				
Standing				
Walking				
Transfers				
Dressing				
Undressing				
Washing				
HABITS: Diet				
Micturition Times Day				
Micturition Times Night				
Defaecation				
DEFECTS OBSERVED: Sores				
Bruises				
Swelling				
Rashes				
				ECC.

This form may be extended by using Nursing Assessment Forms related to specific conditions.

Figure 11.2: West Birmingham Health District — Department of Geriatrics — Habit Retraining Chart

KEY   State of Patient

DRY	= Green Dot
Incontinent of Urine	= Red Dot
Result of Toileting	
Passed Urine in Toilet	= Blue Dot
Not Passed Urine in Toilet	= Yellow Dot
Refused or Absent	= X in Blue

Habit Retraining

Habit retraining, once started, should not be interrupted, as both patient and nurse can be demoralised by failure. Adequate staffing is required, so that the number of patients being retrained must be decided by the head of the team in relation to the number of staff available.

A rigid toiletting regime should not be imposed on patients who are candidates for habit retraining and too frequent emptying of the bladder (more than two-hourly) without adjustments to suit the individual need, may militate against the restoration of continence by reducing the effective capacity of the bladder. Where possible patients should be encouraged to postpone micturition for as long as possible.[1] During the night patients are observed but not disturbed unless incontinence occurs. The incontinent episodes, however, are recorded so that the information can be used to organise a suitable routine to meet the patients' needs.

An Example of Habit Retraining

The example which follows describes the retraining of one particular patient, using the chart. There are a number of different factors affecting bladder behaviour, so although the procedure outlined can be applied generally, the results will not necessarily be the same for other patients.

Day 1. The results of two-hourly observation from 9.0 a.m. until 9.0 p.m. were recorded on the bottom line of the chart. Incontinence occurred at 9.0 a.m., 11.0 a.m., 5.0 p.m. and 7.0 p.m.

Day 3. Adjustments were made at 8.0 a.m., 10.0 a.m., 4.0 p.m. and 6.0 p.m., to enable the patient to void before incontinence occurred. Further study of the chart shows that toiletting time at 1.0 p.m. was continued as the patient voided in the toilet; 3.0 p.m. and 9.0 p.m. were discontinued as the patient did not void. Thus the seven voiding times were reduced to five. The patient was now continent on the following regime: 8.0 a.m., 10.0 a.m., 1.0 p.m., 4.0 p.m., and 6.0 p.m.

Day 6. The two-hourly intervals were extended by half an hour until three-hourly intervals were established.

Day 14. Toiletting had now been reduced to four times daily. Night recordings showed adjustments on similar principles.

Thus through adjustments and extending of voiding times a new pattern of micturition was established which enabled the patient to become continent. The recordings were then discontinued, but a follow-up was carried out from time to time. Extending the intervals between voidings, providing the patient can cope, is of great importance when considering discharge of patients to their own homes or to residential establishments, for obvious practical reasons. The results of two 13-week trials carried out at Dudley Road Hospital, Birmingham, are shown in Table 11.1. The average age of patients was 79.

Table 11.1: Results of Trials at Dudley Road Hospital

No. of patients	Success	Partial	Failed	Died
20 (Male)	12	4	3	1
11 (Female)	8	1	2	0

The charting system, in addition to its use in habit retaining, is also of great value in providing instant information about bladder behaviour to all staff. It can indicate response to treatment, reveal urinary tract abnormalities, is an aid to diagnosis and is the nurse's on-going report. It can also provide information relevant to research. Further information about the chart, with detailed instructions on its use, may be found in a series of articles in the *Nursing Mirror*.[2]

Alternative Nursing Management

When a pattern of micturition does not emerge and habit retraining cannot be carried out, an alternative form of nursing management will be required. This involves a rigid toileting regime and the use of personal protection. The toileting schedule is imposed on the patient until a regular response is established. The procedure must be carefully explained by a senior member of staff, so that the patient (and junior staff) appreciate its necessity.

Where incontinence cannot be managed by this method, Kanga Pants can be used (see Appendix C). They may be used in conjunction with habit retraining, particularly in the early stages before the pattern of micturition has evolved, but their main use is for those patients where habit retraining fails. They are comfortable to wear, and do not induce sweating; some patients with a lesser degree of urinary leakage wear them with success in bed. Kanga Pants are of unique design, in that the patient's skin remains dry. The fabric is 100 per cent polyester which looks and feels like soft cotton lock-knit; it is permeable and non-absorbent, and allows urine to pass through freely while remaining dry itself. There is a waterproof plastic 'marsupial' pouch with a front opening on the outside of the pants, into which is placed a special pad (the Kanga Pad), folded double. These pads are essential, and ordinary incontinence roll should never be substituted. The pad must be changed before saturation and the frequency of changing can be determined by careful checking. The habit retraining chart, with suitable modifications, can be used for this purpose. Kanga Pants must fit like swimming trunks and sizing is by hip measurements. The legs are elasticated and can be adjusted. An important feature is that the pad can be changed without removing the pants.

A careful explanation of the working in principle of Kanga Pants must be given to the patient, who may be understandably reluctant to void urine directly into the pants, and may consequently wish to put the pad next to the skin instead of in the pouch. The nurse will need to support and encourage the patient while this system of management is being established.

Nursing Management in the Community

Although domiciliary nursing resources are different from those in hospital, the habit retraining procedure and the use of alternative nursing management may be practised successfully at home. The right conditions presuppose a co-operative patient with adequate mental resources to make simple recordings on a chart, and with sufficient mobility to be able to visit the lavatory at regular intervals or, if Kanga Pants are being used, to be able to change the pads. During the initial stages a community nurse should be available to supervise whichever procedure is being followed. With progress the visits can be reduced, except for regular follow-up visits to ensure that continence is maintained. If a patient lives alone with no supportive relative or friend, short-term admission to hospital for initial assessment may be advisable. After successful rehabilitation, and prior to discharge, the home conditions should be assessed and the necessary support services organised.

Rehabilitative Nursing in the Community – A New Development

In one area of Birmingham, where shortage of nursing staff in the community nursing service poses a problem, a hospital-based team of three nurses has been set up in order to carry out rehabilitative nursing of incontinent elderly patients at home. Funding is from the Department of Geriatric Medicine at Dudley Road Hospital. The nursing team was carefully selected and trained (for six weeks) and given supervised clinical practice on the wards. Apart from the valuable service which this team is providing for the patients, it is extending its special skills, as practised in hospital, to the community nurse. Closer liaison between hospital and community services is also resulting. Evaluations in 1978 and 1979 have shown a considerable degree of success; out of 55 patients, 34 were habit retrained and 12 enabled to use Kanga Pants effectively. Following these evaluations it has been decided that all community nurses in the area should receive training in this type of management. In teamwork of this kind, achievement rests very much upon the qualities of the team leader, and the calibre of the nurses.

Notes

1. Willington, F.L. (1978), 'Urinary Incontinence and Urgency', *Practitioner*, *220*, 739-47.
2. Clay, E.C. (1978), 'Incontinence of Urine', *Nursing Mirror* (March 2, 9, 16 and 23).

12 A BEHAVIOURAL APPROACH TO THE MANAGEMENT OF INCONTINENCE IN THE ELDERLY

R.K. Turner

Introduction

The next decade will see a very considerable increase in the proportion of the population that is over retiring age. Questions about the actual pattern of caring are beyond the scope of this chapter; on the other hand, anyone who is interested in the improvement of actual facilities for the aged can hardly avoid the problem of incontinence.

Failure of sphincter control is one of the major reasons for the admission of elderly people into long-stay beds in hospital. It would be very easy to regret the inability and unwillingness of families to cope with incontinent relatives; but these patients are also shunned by professional caregivers. Nowhere is there reluctance to tolerate incontinence more evident than in the policy of many residential homes to refuse admission to old people who are incontinent or who have a history of unreliable bladder or bowel control (see Chapter 13). This can be especially unfair when an occasional bed wet is enshrined in the patient's notes as 'incontinence', even though such accidents have been recorded only during illness or under the stress of admission to hospital.

Undoubtedly, it is often difficult to adopt a therapeutic attitude towards an incontinent patient, especially if the client is also unco-operative and uncommunicative. However, incontinence may often be attributed to the ward or home environment. For example, an elderly patient with urgency of micturition may be unable to get quickly enough to the toilet or commode due to difficulty in rising from a poorly-designed chair; the height of the patient's bed may be a critical factor, responsible for nocturnal enuresis if the patient cannot get out of bed without assistance and no night staff are available. Such incidents as these may well be the first step to the labelling of a patient as 'incontinent'. Then again, staff of wards with demented and confused patients sometimes recount how a particular patient urinates in the fire-bucket or some other receptacle; but toilets are often poorly signposted and sometimes they are really quite difficult to find. Accordingly, it is of interest that the authors of an American research study reported that painting a line from the day room to the toilets brought about a very considerable reduction in the incontinence of two patients.[1] Other examples can be found where incontinence is significantly reduced by relatively simple alterations in the patient's environment.

Good nursing practice requires the regular changing of soiled clothing and this can soon become a highly regimented toiletting of all patients in an attempt to 'catch' the errant bowel or bladder before an accident occurs. There are two weaknesses in this common nursing practice. First, it assumes that all patients can be treated as a group; yet, there is considerable variation as regards the pattern of bladder and bowel functioning. The absurdity of this assumption is apparent if we consider what would be the reaction of normal adults if they were expected to visit the toilet at specific times of the day and night. Secondly, the 'wet-round' can easily become a never-ending routine; the last patient is no sooner dry and clean than the whole process has to begin again, proceeding inexorably through day and night. Seen from the point of view of the patient, individual attention of staff may be available only during the wet-round or on those occasions when the patient has had an accident and requires a change of clothing. It is under such circumstances that behaviour therapy has some insights to offer to the management of the elderly and incontinent patient. Behaviour therapy leads to the very careful examination of the simple question: to what extent is the incontinence avoidable by changing the way in which staff and relatives deal with the patient?

Behaviour Therapy

The behavioural approach has provided a practical means for improving the social behaviour of long-stay elderly patients:[2] for example, studies have demonstrated increased physical and recreational activity[3, 4] and reinstated verbal behaviour.[5] Although there is, admittedly, only a fairly small literature on it, behaviour therapy suggests new ways of tackling some very common problems that face those who have to design services for the aged.

There have been few attempts to treat incontinence in the elderly by behavioural techniques. But, there is a wealth of evidence that similar methods are effective *and* feasible for the treatment of children with disorders of sphincter control. For example, day wetting and soiling as well as nighttime wetting of the bed have been tackled very successfully by clinicians using behaviour therapy.[6-10] The same methods of treatment have also proved to be effective in the management of incontinence amongst residents in hospitals for the mentally handicapped.[11, 12]

The aim of the behavioural approach is to provide an opportunity for the patient to learn more appropriate behaviour. Of course, the problem with the elderly is more a matter of helping the patient to relearn old skills that have been lost through physical illness or in the confusion and disorientation of the ageing process.

Physical maturation sets the limits as regards the speed with which children become toilet-trained. Similarly, the possibility of retraining sphincter control in the elderly patient is limited by the degree of organic pathology. Clearly, this chapter is concerned more with those cases in whom incontinence occurs despite the apparent capacity of the patient to regain control. The design of exercises to retrain the relevant musculature lies more appropriately within the province of the physio-therapist; behaviour therapy suggests how to assess and then to modify the patient's capacity and motivation to regain continence. Willington[13] has drawn on Pavlovian conditioning principles as a basis for habit retraining; the purpose of this chapter is to broaden the theoretical framework by incorporating the findings of behavioural approaches which emphasise the environmental determinants of abnormal behaviour.

Behavioural Assessment

Just as in good nursing practice, the first step in setting up a behavioural treatment is to make a careful recording of the patient's normal pattern of micturition and defecation. This pre-treatment record should include such information as the times when the patient urinates or defecates. In the search for the patient's habitual pattern of, say, bladder functioning, it may also be useful to ask about the patient's pattern of micturition under normal circumstances (e.g. at home). It is essential to enquire about the consequences for the patient of the incontinence. How do staff or relatives deal with the problem behaviour and what are the consequences of the patient being wet or soiled? Finally, what are the antecedents of the behaviour? For example, does the incontinence usually follow a meal, or is it determined by some apparent time cycle? Does the incontinence always occur when a particular nurse is on duty or when grandchildren are visiting the family at home?

Several methods of recording incontinence have been described for general application in nursing[13, 14] (see Chapter 11). Clearly, the exact form of a chart will vary according to staff and other considerations;

but, the essential features of a behavioural record are summarised in Table 12.1 under headings of the antecedents of behaviour, the behaviour itself and its consequences.

Table 12.1: The ABC of Recording Behaviour

*A*ntecedent events

What seems to set the stage for the patient's incontinence?

For example — after a meal
— time of day
— when someone has forgotten to prompt the patient
— after some 'stressful' event (e.g. visitors)
— when a particular member of staff is on duty
— patient is on the way to toilet
— location

*B*ehaviour

Describe the problem behaviour
— is it incontinence of micturition, faeces, or both?
— frequency per day or some appropriate time period
— where does it occur (e.g. in clothing)?
— is it a full bladder discharge, or dribbling?
— is it a full motion passed, smear?

*C*onsequences

(1) What are the social consequences (for the patient) of the incontinence?
— how is it handled?
— what is said to the patient?
— does the patient help to clean up soiled clothing, etc?
(2) What are the consequences of the patient being continent?
— is the patient encouraged and praised for any attempt at voluntary control of sphincter?
— is any success recognised by staff or is it ignored?

Having defined the problem behaviour, the next step is to agree on appropriate goals for treatment. Both these aspects of planning need to take into account limitations of the client (e.g. degree of comprehension, memory, co-operation, organic pathology) and environmental restrictions (e.g. staffing level, expectations of staff).

Wherever possible, the patient must be fully involved in the process of assessment *and* the planning of treatment. After all, the success of therapy will be mainly determined by the co-operation of the patient. The patient's motivation to become continent is as crucial in behaviour therapy as in any other treatment.

The management of severely-dementing patients may be aided very significantly even if retraining only helps them to give warning to staff or relatives of their need for bladder evacuation. Accordingly, it would be inappropriate to judge behavioural casework solely by its success in bringing about the complete arrest of incontinence in all cases. The behavioural assessment must set realistic goals, taking into account the effects of severe dementia, social independence and memory disabilities.

Toilet Training

Learning may be defined as a relatively permanent change in behaviour resulting from experience or practice. At a reflex level it is possible to acquire new responses by classical conditioning, but human behaviour is the result of more complex learning processes, as is apparent from the toilet training of children. The first requirement is that the child has attained adequate neural maturation for the development of voluntary bowel and bladder control. Although the exact processes of continence development are still not fully understood, we can speculate that a conditioning process provides the basis for the child's development of the skill of identifying correctly the internal signals that indicate a filling bladder or full rectum; in addition the child must be able to inhibit micturition or defaecation until excretion can occur in a socially approved place.[15]

Anyone who has brought up children will be aware that the processes by which a child becomes toilet-trained involve also a great deal of social learning. The child imitates other children or parents and in this way learns where it is permissible to excrete and the appropriate posture to adopt. Children are also praised by parents for progress towards continence; and of course, there are other occasions when parental disapproval and punishment aids the process of discriminating where the discharge of bowel or bladder is unacceptable. However, our understanding of learning is still incomplete unless we acknowledge that learning is best achieved if broken up into small steps; children have to go through several intermediate steps before they are fully continent. For example, they may need assistance at first in unfastening clothing; they learn gradually to be able to inhibit micturition for increasingly longer periods of time.

To sum up, the learning of the skills that are the basis of continence may be analysed under three main headings. First, there is the element of reflex, respondent conditioning which explains how the individual acquires and then maintains appropriate inhibitory control over sphincters. Secondly, social learning occurs by which we are responsive to the influence of others in the environment, exerted in particular by the rewards that follow success in maintaining continence and the disapproval that is expressed if accidents occur. Thirdly, learning is most efficient if broken into small steps leading to full continence.

The analysis of how children learn to control their sphincters provides a theoretical framework for understanding how best to retrain continence in elderly patients. Admittedly, it would be naive to draw too fixed an analogy and much research is required before we will understand how the process of retraining sphincter control differs from what is experienced in childhood, but at least the framework provides some useful guidelines about factors that are likely to be of significance.

Techniques for Behavioural Treatment of Incontinence

The Alarm Device

This is designed to provide an opportunity for the patient to learn once again to discriminate during sleep a level of bladder volume and pressure that is below the level of automatic discharge. This well-tried technique may be used with the elderly patient who suffers from persistent nightwetting. Figure 12.1 shows diagramatically how the alarm is placed on the patient's bed. The procedure of treatment is relatively straightforward. As soon as the patient wets the bed, the alarm is triggered by the urine-sensitive pads. The patient must then go immediately to the toilet (or use a urine bottle) before returning to sleep. Although the method seems relatively straightforward there are several basic requirements if it is to be clinically effective.[16] First, it is well known from its use with children that the equipment must be designed according to DHSS safety standards in order to avoid buzzer ulcers.[17] Secondly, treatment requires close supervision and particular attention should be paid to the patient who feels humiliated by having to use an alarm that seems to turn a nocturnal accident into a very public event. Finally, there is the obvious point that the patient (as well as the relatives and nursing staff) has to understand how the equipment works and the aims of treatment. The patient must be able to wake up sufficiently to urinate in a commode or at the toilet as soon as the alarm has been triggered by the onset of wetting. Treatment may well need the careful supervision of night-staff or relatives if it is to be effective; this is especially necessary if the patient is a heavy sleeper.

It would be very difficult to use an alarm device for the treatment of daytime wetting without careful modification; the equipment would

Figure 12.1: The 'Bell and Pad' Enuresis Alarm Device

THE "BELL & PAD" ENURESIS ALARM DEVICE.

The diagrams below show you how to make up the bed.

G – TOP DRAW SHEET.
F – BED MAT (GAUZE).
E – ½ DRAW (SEPARATION) SHEET.
D – BED MAT (GAUZE).
C – RUBBER SHEET.
B – MATTRESS.
A – BED.

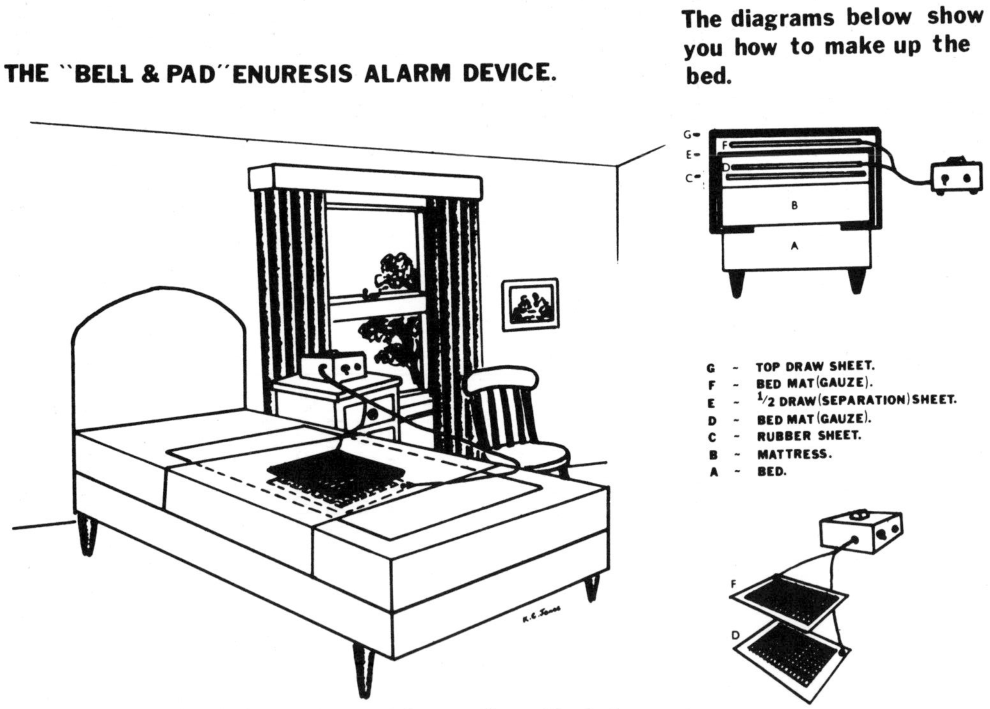

Source: Reproduced with the permission of Crescent Press, Birmingham.

have to be very small and it is not usually practical to use an auditory signal to alert the patient after wetting. Millard[18] used faradic stimulation in the treatment of a stress-incontinence patient, but such an approach seeems unacceptable with elderly patients. One possibility that merits further research evaluation is the use of a radio transmitter device; the equipment is very small and can be worn discreetly under clothing without causing embarrassment to the patient. As soon as the patient begins to urinate, a radio signal is emitted which can be picked up by a wireless receiver; this enables staff (or relatives) to take the patient to the toilet immediately. Certainly such a device would have several applications, ranging from the monitoring of bladder functioning in ambulatory patients to the development of treatment programmes with day-wetting elderly patients. This type of equipment is a direct derivative of toilet training apparatus that has been developed for use with young children, as also in the training of the mentally handicapped. However, the method has still to be evaluated in clinical trials to test its effectiveness and feasibility when used with aged patients.

Of course, equipment such as this could be adapted so that the patient is alerted by a tactile or mild faradic stimulus immediately after the onset of micturition. The method would then be similar to bio-feedback techniques that facilitate the development of the voluntary control of physiological responses in patients (e.g. bio-feedback techniques for control of hypertension, migraine and epilepsy). In this respect the method has some similarity to attempts to retain recto-sphincteric responses in patients with faecal incontinence[19] as well as clinical studies of pessary devices in stress incontinent women.

Behaviour Modification

An alarm device teaches the patient improved self-control. However, just as toilet training of children depends on social learning, so also behaviour modification emphasises the role played by the environment in maintaining continence. That is to say, the behavioural approach examines how staff and relatives respond to the patient. The guiding principle is that desirable behaviour should be rewarded while the frequency of inappropriate behaviour can be reduced by changing its consequences (e.g. ignoring it, showing disapproval).

The emphasis is on the environmental determinants of problem behaviour and the aim of treatment is expressed always in terms of specifying what is desired behaviour (e.g. dry and/or clean pants when checked periodically by day or night).

There have been many techniques which may be summarised under the headings of behaviour modification. All have in common, however, their use of what is called 'reinforcement'. This usually refers to a reward whose effect is to increase the behaviour that follows. For example, if a patient is praised and has the undivided attention of staff when dry, then this is a reinforcer.

The aim of any effective plan must be to ensure that the patient is given ample rewards for being clean and dry. The baseline record chart provides a way of examining how the patient's environment is maintaining the incontinence. For many patients who live in a crowded ward (or indeed at home with busy relatives), one of the few times they receive attention is after an 'accident'. Even though the resulting interchange between patient and staff may often sound like a reprimand, nevertheless it is still attention. The purpose of the behavioural assessment is to examine what effect the incontinence has on the patient's interaction with others; the next step is to modify the interaction so that attention and perhaps more specific rewards *follow* continence. Reward is then contingent upon desired rather than undesired behaviour. Admittedly, a behavioural treatment plan attempts to modify behaviour by introducing very specific and controlled contingent reinforcement. However, it is assumed that this contrived system gives way to the natural reinforcement that occurs when staff encourage continence, and the patient's level of self-esteem is raised.

But, first it is necessary to find out what *are* appropriate rewards for the individual patient. It is all very well to state that a patient will work towards the goal of continence if rewarded with staff atttention or cigarettes. But, it is a big assumption that staff attention *is* welcome to the patient; it may well be the case that the opportunity to have a five minute chat or a game of cards is rewarding only if it is with a particular member of staff or relative. Similarly, cigarettes may not be as rewarding to the patient as the chance to watch a particular programme on TV. Another crucial requirement is that the reward comes as soon as possible after the desired behaviour: rewarding the patient for being continent is unlikely to be effective if it is delayed to such an extent that the patient has forgotten; this may be an even more crucial consideration when patients suffer from poor memory.

The behavioural assessment must also identify relevant environmental restrictions. If shortages of staff are such that few patients can have the undivided attention of a single member of staff for ten minutes, then a programme that rewards the patient with staff attention is likely to lead to very considerable problems on the ward as a whole. It is very important to discuss with all concerned the demands that treatment will make on their time; undoubtedly, the advantages of a patient being clean and dry can be outweighed by the disadvantages of changing the normal pattern of a whole household or a complete ward. Acceptance of incontinence by staff or relatives *may well outweigh* advantages to be gained from a treatment programme especially if it necessitates radical changes in the normal routine of a ward or household.

A systematic manipulation of rewards so that desired behaviour (i.e. continence) is reinforced, instead of the undesired incontinence, is a very constructive approach to training. Such a form of modification is even more effective if 'shaped' so that the patient is rewarded for each 'small step'. However, it is clear from the training of continence in the young that it is sometimes facilitated by some aversive reinforcement. If the aim is to decrease the frequency of undesirable behaviour then it is either no longer followed by reinforcement *or* its consequences are unpleasant to the learner. The careful combination of these two aspects of learning are carefully balanced in behaviour modification programmes.

Atthowe[20] set up a special therapeutic programme for the treatment of twelve patients who were enuretic at night. The cases had lived in psychiatric institutions for over 20 years; half the patients had been lobotomised and they were all described as being delusional and generally uncommunicative. The therapists exerted some fairly strong social pressures on patients not to be incontinent. The patients were placed in a crowded ward, but with patients who were, for the most part, continent; whenever one of the incontinent patients was wet at night, then the wetting caused considerable inconvenience for the whole ward. On four occasions during the night the enuretic patients were escorted to the toilet where they were detained for ten minutes irrespective of whether or not they had been found to be wet. The social pressure on the patients to become dry was exerted through that part of the programme which required that all the other patients in the ward were also wakened at the same time on these four occasions of toiletting. This 'aversive' routine was maintained for a total of two months before a reward system was introduced; this involved tokens which could be used to 'buy' better sleeping quarters. These tokens were given to the incontinent patients as an immediate reward for each night they were recorded as having been dry; additionally, some of the nocturnal visits to the toilet were phased out progressively as the patient became dry. When a patient had been dry for a whole week he was allowed to sleep undisturbed through the whole night and later was given the opportunity to move to what was described as better sleeping quarters.

One can question both the efficacy and the ethics of some aspects of the treatment routine, but it is of interest that the patients did become dry under this regime. During the two month aversive regime all but the most severely enuretic of the patients ceased to wet the bed. Furthermore, after six months of the reward programme all the patients had become dry at night and this progress was maintained over a 43-month period of follow-up.

There are several things of interest in this study, although it is admittedly hard to see how its replication could be justified in the setting of a British NHS hospital. First, the reward system was more effective than the first part of the programme when patients were subjected to a really strongly punitive regime that exerted massive social pressure. Secondly, even allowing for the small number of patients it is of interest that these results were obtained with an extreme sample of chronic patients with a very considerable degree of physical organic pathology.

Hartie and Black[21] describe the results of a reinforcement programme, designed to reduce nocturnal enuresis in long-stay and aged patients. The study concerned only five patients who were members of a 45-bedded long-stay ward. The programme began with a one-month period of observation when the frequency of wetting was recorded on charts. In the treatment phase of the study, each patient was reminded to urinate before going to bed. The night staff were also told to raise the patient if awake one hour after going to bed and then again at 2.0 a.m. Rewards were given the next morning by night staff to all who had been dry during the night at the time of the bed check at 7.0 a.m. Day staff were also asked to praise each patient for success in remaining dry. The authors emphasise that the reward was decided on an individual basis, in each case after careful discussion with the patient. The authors present only a fairly brief description of their results, but their case data suggest that the rates of nocturnal enuresis showed a progressive reduction over the two-month period when the study was in force. Also, the improvement was maintained in follow-up. However, none of the patients attained a period of complete continence.

Pollock and Liberman[1] describe the results of a study of the treatment of five demented men who were incontinent of urine. All were patients on a geriatric unit; also, the patients were all described as having a diagnosis of chronic organic brain syndrome.

Patients were given a two-hourly pants check during the baseline, treatment phase of the programme. The treatment phase was in two parts. For a period of one week, the patients had to mop up their own incontinence and they were not changed unless they requested it specifically. There then followed a three-week period during which patients were also given a reward (cigarette or sweet) as well as a few minutes of conversation following each occasion when they were found to be dry at a check of clothing.

The results were negative in so far as three patients improved (no data are given), but in two cases the condition deteriorated. This is a difficult study to evaluate, not the least because in at least one patient the deterioration was very marked, yet the authors attributed it to a change in medication. Also, the authors commented that the giving of reinforcement was variable. In at least one patient there was a massive improvement after the study was completed; he was given cigarettes for being dry at each check of clothing, but the authors observed that the improvement also coincided with the arrival on the ward of new female staff.

The authors also describe how two patients were unable to find their way to the toilet. A white line was painted on the floor from the day room to the toilet and this was said to help one of their patients though not the most severe. The authors were correct in emphasising that it would have been more appropriate to reward patients for the 'small steps' they made towards becoming continent; for example, by prompting a patient and then rewarding him for getting nearer each day to the toilet before having an accident.

Conclusions

All research reports on the management of incontinence, irrespective of any particular theoretical viewpoint, emphasise the importance of adequate incentives for staff or relatives to co-operate.[22] Incontinence is very difficult to manage; it can all too easily be interpreted by staff or relatives as an almost hostile act, directed by the patient against them. Indeed, it is very common for incontinence to be attributed to laziness; it is then difficult to convince staff and relatives that the problem *is* remediable. Plans to ensure that patients are rewarded for improved sphincter control will fail if the staff are not themselves praised and encouraged. In setting up any procedure to improve the management of incontinence the key first step is to ensure that staff or relatives are themselves fully in the picture as to the aims and methods of treatment. Otherwise, it is very easy for the 'new' management of incontinence to be construed as an implicit criticism of what may have been accepted previously as good management.

Economic considerations should be enough to convince those at management level in nursing or social services that it is worth doing something to reduce the level of incontinence. Laundry costs alone are high and may be reduced by new initiatives in management[23] (see Chapters 9, 10 and 11). In addition there are indirect benefits of allowing nursing staff more time to devote to rewarding interaction with patients. The improved self-esteem in patients is likely to be, by far, the single most important outcome of any significant reduction in incontinence.

Behaviour therapy for incontinence has been evaluated in so few studies that we have still to draw upon the evidence of its efficiency with children and young adults. Accordingly, it is premature to lay claim for the feasibility and effectiveness of this approach with elderly people. The main advantage is that it offers staff and relatives a systematic analysis of the training of continence.

The behavioural approach has originated from careful experimental studies of how we learn. Behaviour therapy must be distinguished from the traditional viewpoint that prevails in psychological medicine; there is no gainsaying that incontinence can be attributable to organic pathology, in many cases, and dementia is undoubtedly a very significant factor. However, when physical approaches to treatment have been tried without success, nursing staff or relatives are still left with a patient who wets or soils clothing and bedding. Talking-based pscyhotherapies have little to offer by way of clear guidelines for what can actually be done to help the patient and some form of training is manifestly appropriate.

There is a wealth of evidence that nocturnal enuresis can be reduced very significantly in younger age groups using the alarm method. This well-tried technique offers a systematic means of retraining the patient to tolerate increased bladder volume without automatic discharge. Future studies are required when the method has been evaluated over a period of more than eight weeks.[24] A urine detector based on the same design but suitably adapted offers a practical way of observing bladder functioning during the daytime; it remains to be seen whether such an approach might be used to arrest diurnal urinary incontinence. At present the equipment would seem to be of most use in the careful observation of daytime bladder functioning in ambulatory elderly patients.

The environmental determinants of incontinence are not fully understood; and yet, it is apparent from differences between different wards of the same hospital with fairly similar patients[25] that patients do seem to respond to particular staff, regimes and so on. We still do not know why there should be such variation. All we can deduce is that the patient's environment *is* relevant if we are to understand why someone is incontinent.

Accordingly, the behavioural method offers a systematic way to analyse what it is that contributes to the incontinence. The evidence of an admittedly small number of studies suggests that the overall level of incontinence in chronic patients can be reduced through a systematic ward programme. But, again, success seems to have been achieved by implementing a surprisingly punitive regime in one American study. It remains to be seen whether programmes can be similarly successful where the emphasis is more upon reward and positive reinforcement; the limited evidence of the one study by Atthowe[20] certainly did suggest that reward was better than the punishing routine that was used in the American project.

Indications for Research

Incontinence is so common among our elderly population that research is required which is other than the purely medical (e.g. into surgical or drug techniques). Careful evaluation of different management routines as well as the improvement of nursing aids are both required urgently. The behavioural framework offers the very significant advantage that both the theory and the methodology have already been well-tried with other age groups.

First, research is needed to develop improved charting methods for monitoring incontinence. Ideally, it should be possible to monitor a patient's bladder functioning so that information is available about the individual, characteristic pattern of bladder discharge. Surgical and traditional methods of investigation are intrusive (not to say unpleasant) and there would seem to be a lot to be said for observation methods which provide information about bladder functioning less directly (e.g. urine detectors that can be used with ambulatory patients).

When we turn our attention to actual methods of treatment, it is important to determine the limits of behaviour therapy. For example, is it possible to retrain continence (either bladder or bowel) in the presence of severe dementia? Then again, it may well be the case that there are different stages of dementia, and continence may be retrained to a varying extent, depending upon the degree of dementia. Certainly, the reduction of incontinence may well be a qualified but significant success even if continence is not regained totally. Nocturnal incontinence in the absence of demonstrable organic, daytime incontinence is a very real problem which causes considerable social distress. It remains to be seen whether such cases respond to behaviour therapy. Perhaps, generalisation of bladder control from day to night-time sphincter control might be found, as seems likely when children are treated who experience day and night-time wetting.[26]

It may be feasible for behaviour therapists to improve incontinence in severely confused and disorientated patients by increasing environmental cues which act to remind constantly and appropriately the patient of the need to urinate. Systematic studies of learning and a consistent model of how continence is achieved provide a firm basis for the in-service training of staff and additional support for relatives. It is to be hoped that very specific studies of behaviour therapy for incontinence in the elderly are complemented by similar attention paid to the best way to organise in-service staff training and increased support for the relatives.

Notes

1. Pollock, D.D. and Liberman, R.P. (1974), 'Behaviour Therapy of Incontinence in Demented Inpatients', *Gerontologist, 14*, 488-91.

2. Mumford, S. and Carpenter, G. (1979), 'Psychological Services and the Elderly', *Bull. Brit. Psych. Soc., 32*, 286-8.

3. Jenkins, J., Felce, D., Lunt, B. and Powell, L. (1977), 'Increasing Engagement in Activity of Residents in Old People's Homes by Providing Recreational Materials', *Behav. Res. and Therapy, 15*, 429-34.

4. Libb, J.W. and Clements, C.B. (1969), 'Token Reinforcement in an Exercise Programme for Hospitalised Patients', *Perceptual and Motor Skills, 28*, 957-8.

5. Hoyer, W.J., Kafer, R.A. and Simpson, S.C. (1974), 'Reinstatement of Verbal Behaviour in Elderly Mental Patients Using Operant Procedures', *Gerontologist, 14*, 149-52.

6. Ashkenasky, Z. (1975), 'The Treatment of Encropresis Using a Discriminative Stimulus and Positive Reinforcement', *J. Behav. Therapy & Exper. Psychiatry, 6*, 155-7.

7. Slukin, A. (1975), 'Encopresis: A Behavioural Approach Described', *Social Work Today, 5*, 643-6.

8. Turner, R.K. (1973), 'Conditioning Treatment of Nocturnal Enuresis: Present Status' in Kolvin, I., MacKeith, R.C. and Meadows, S.R. (eds.), *Bladder Control and Enuresis* (SIMP/Heinemann, London).

9. Turner, R.K. and Taylor, P.D. (1974), 'Conditioning Treatment of Nocturnal Enuresis in Adults: Preliminary Findings', *Behav. Res. and Therapy, 12*, 273-8.

10. Doleys, D.M. (1977), 'Behavioural Treatments for Nocturnal Enuresis in

Children: A Review of the Recent Literature', *Psychol. Bull., 84*, 30-54.
11. Azrin, N.H. and Foxx, R.M. (1971), 'A Rapid Method of Toilet Training the Institutionalised Retarded', *J. Applied Behav. Anal., 4*, 89-99.
12. Smith, P.S., Britton, P.G., Johnson, M. and Thomas, D.A. (1975), 'Problems Involved in Toilet Training Profoundly Mentally Handicapped Children', *Behav. Res. and Therapy, 13*, 301-8.
13. Willington, F.L. (1976), 'The Physiological Basis of Retraining for Continence', in Willington, F.L. (ed.), *Incontinence in the Elderly* (Academic Press, London).
14. Clay, E.C. (1978), 'Incontinence of Urine', *Nursing Mirror* (9 March), 36-8.
15. Meadows, R., MacKeith, R. and Turner, R.K. (1973), 'How Children Become Dry' in Kolvin, I., MacKeith, R. and Meadows, S.R. (eds.), *Bladder Control and Enuresis* (SIMP/Heinemann, London).
16. Notes on the treatment procedure have been prepared and may be obtained from the author on request.
17. Dische, S. (1973), 'Treatment of Enuresis with an Enuresis Alarm' in Kolvin, I., MacKeith, R.C. and Meadows, S.R. (eds.) *Bladder Control and Enuresis* (SIMP/Heinemann, London).
18. Millard, D.W. (1966), 'A Conditioning Treatment for "Giggle" Micturition', *Behav. Res. and Therapy, 4*, 229-31.
19. Engel, B.T., Nikoomanesh, P.S. and Schuster, M.M. (1974), 'Operant Conditioning of Recto-sphincteric Responses in the Treatment of Fecal Incontinence', *New Eng. J. Med., 290*, 646-9.
20. Atthowe, J.M. (1972), 'Controlling Nocturnal Enuresis in Severely Disabled and Chronic Patients', *Behav. Therapy, 3*, 232-9.
21. Hartie, A. and Black, D. (1975), 'A Dry Bed is the Objective', *Nursing Times* (November), 1874-6.
22. Maney, J.Y. (1976), 'A Behavioural Therapy Approach to Bladder Retraining', *Nurs. Clin. North America, 11*, 179-88.
23. Tam, G., Knox, J.G. and Adamson, M. (1978), 'A Cost-effectiveness Trial of Incontinence Pants', *Nursing Times* (20 July), 1198-200.
24. Collins, R.W. and Plaska, T. (1975), 'Mourer's Conditioning Treatment for Enuresis Applied to Geriatric Residents of a Nursing Home', *Behav. Therapy, 6*, 632-8.
25. Corp, M. and Turner, R.K. (1978), 'A Survey of Nurse Attitudes to Incontinence; A Summary of Findings', unpublished manuscript.
26. Jehu, D., Morgan, R.T.T., Turner, R.K. and Jones, A. (1977), 'A Controlled Trial of the Treatment of Nocturnal Enuresis in Residential Homes for Children', *Behav. Res. and Therapy, 15*, 1-16.

13 THE ROLE OF THE SOCIAL SERVICES

Julia Taylor

Introduction

In the context of the complex personal and family problems which are presented to the social services departments, incontinence appears as one of the highly emotive aspects of human behaviour around which the threat of breakdown in goodwill tends to focus. In the midst of multiple difficulties, lack of control of bowel and bladder functions can become the 'last straw' for families and friends who are trying to help, and can at times be perceived as deliberately provocative behaviour, where relationships are already under stress. The incontinent person is therefore likely to be 'at risk', in the sense that he might forfeit the goodwill of those upon whom he is dependent for his well-being. A range of concealed emotions might be projected into those that are expressed about the incontinence. It can be relatively more acceptable, for example, to express rejection because of 'dirty' bowel and bladder functions, than rejection of the person because there has been long-standing disenchantment with him generally. Rejection, or withdrawal of goodwill, can be experienced at the hands of professional helpers as well as of families. Taboos and inhibitions connected with bodily functions in our society influence behaviour and attitudes generally, and people are involved in providing personal help and support to incontinent people on a professional basis are not free from the impact of the prevailing culture.

The effort to help effectively with the management and reversal of a pattern of incontinence, and at the same time to work through the many other difficulties that might be presented, calls for a high level of professional competence, self-awareness and ability to work in close co-operation, not only with the client and his family, but with colleagues within and without the social services department.

The Nature of the Social Services' Response

Social services departments undertake responsibilities that are determined by legislation and when considering the part that can be played

220

in the amelioration of problems arising from incontinence, it is important to recognise the scope and limitations. Broadly speaking, social services departments carry a range of responsibilities in respect of certain vulnerable people throughout the life-span: children, young people and families at risk; the mentally ill; the mentally handicapped; the physically handicapped; and elderly people at risk. The broad aim of intervention is to overcome difficulties that have threatened adequate functioning, or resulted in breakdown. Incontinence might be one of the major management problems presented by mentally and/or physically handicapped children and adults, placing them at risk of a breakdown in their overall management within their families. Enuresis might be the factor creating a high degree of risk for the child in a tense and vulnerable family. Stress within the family might be a contributing factor to the child's enuresis. In old age, incontinence might jeopardise the elderly person's chances of continuing to live in the place of his choice whether that be in his own home, with his family, in sheltered housing or in a residential home.

The philosophy of the Seebohm Report, which was reflected in the Local Government Social Services Act 1970, was to strengthen the capacity of the family and the community to respond to the needs of the more vulnerable members of society. Mental and physical ill-health, handicap or frailty, emotional deprivation and stress, poor financial, social and environmental factors, all undermine the capacity to manage daily life adequately in an increasingly competitive society. Incontinence might be a very significant factor in the lives of some of these vulnerable people, and it is within the comprehensive effort to support clients and their families and to help them to manage their day to day lives successfully, that social services departments will participate in the effort to relieve the problem posed by incontinence. Where it is clear that the family does not have the capacity to cope, or where there is no family and no family substitute, where the client cannot be helped to manage independently, and where no other resource is appropriate, social services' residential homes might be looked to, in order to meet the need. When this ensues, it is important that the residential staff have the ability and the resources with which to provide an effective response to incontinence.

Staff and Settings

Social services deploy staff with particular skills and functions in a range of settings. There is likely to be a variety of ways in which incontinence is encountered and worked with therefore, and it is by no means the field social worker's involvement that is representative of social services' effort to provide help. The most usual settings in which social services staff are at work are as follows:

Domiciliary (including sheltered housing)
Hospitals (all departments)
Residential homes
Day centres (all client groups)
Adult training centres
Children's centres (day nurseries).

The personnel most usually deployed by social services departments are:

Social workers
Social work assistants/aides
Occupational therapists
Home helps (together with home-help organisers, home care officers)
Good neighbours
Night sitters
Family aides
Day centre organisers and assistants
Children's centre organisers and assistants
Hospital social workers
Residential social workers
Care assistants
Domestic workers
Foster parents
Volunteers recruited and deployed by social services departments in all settings.

It is probably clear from a consideration of the variety of settings and personnel that there are numerous points at which incontinence can be encountered as a feature of a client's difficulties and management problems. The extremely varied qualifications, experience, and skills of the personnel involved pose a challenge to social services departments: first to agree and set out clear policies in respect of incontinence, that staff can implement throughout the service; secondly to ensure adequate, appropriate training programmes for all staff in relation to this aspect of their work; and finally to negotiate and ensure the necessary co-operation with health service colleagues, at all levels, in the work undertaken by social services personnel in relation to the management of incontinence.

Establishing the Basis for Good Practice

With such a diversity of roles, functions, responsibilities, training and experience within social services departments, it is only to be expected that there will be a subtle variety of perceptions of incontinence and that these differing perceptions will influence the responses that are thought appropriate and necessary. Amongst the professional helpers, there still remains some likelihood that incontinent people will be subjected at times to extremely insensitive attitudes and behaviour, which negates any genuine effort to help in the true sense. Professional social work is one of the 'core' activities of social services departments, and the essential principles upon which it rests can be of value in enabling social services departments to establish the attitudes, skills and other resources that are required in working with incontinent clients, in whatever setting.

Social work is a problem-solving process. Incontinence should always be viewed as posing real problems to the person who is experiencing it. The process of solving the problem should be given careful consideration. Acceptance that incontinence inevitably accompanies disability, handicap and old age should be resisted.

Social work practice draws on what is known about human growth and development in an effort to understand reactions to stress and deprivation, and to develop awareness and understanding of how people might be enabled to develop the capacity to overcome difficulties and setbacks. It is important that social services department staff, particularly those who are closely involved with helping clients with the management of bowel and bladder functions, should understand the way in which sphincter control is established and the anxiety that centres around acquiring a high measure of control in early life in our society. The causes and effects of loss of sphincter control need to be understood by social services department staff in order that they may be able to question appropriately and assess the sequence of events in their clients' lives. By questioning and developing understanding, the strategy whereby incontinence is overcome can begin to emerge. Thoughtful consideration and use of the available theory strengthen the development of a professional approach to the management of incontinence and help to dispel the more personal reactions of anger, frustration or revulsion. This is of real importance to staff who are most frequently on the receiving end. Care assistants or home-helps can be personally affronted by it and feel that 'it was done on purpose, to spite me'. The same reaction is frequently voiced by clients' families. In the effort to ensure the maintenance of families' understanding and goodwill it is important that social services department personnel can constructively pursue the expression of feeling such as this.

Fundamental to social work practice is the attitude that respects and values the individual and that aims to safeguard the right of the individual to determine his own goals. The right to self-determination is difficult to establish, and is affected by constraints at the best of times. People who have the disadvantage of handicap, frailty and deprivation are at risk of being seen as less eligible in the struggle to achieve personally-determined goals. Where incontinence is a feature of disability, it seems essential that social services departments ensure that clients' self-esteem is strengthened or restored as a result of the interaction with staff, and that the right to make choices and decisions is also upheld. A poor self-image and lack of spontaneity, which indicates low morale, are frequently associated with incontinence.

In offering help with a view to reversing a pattern of incontinence, social work principles would suggest that it is necessary 'to start where the client is'. In other words, it is essential to know how the client sees things. What constraints exist for him? What does he want to do? What can he do? What does he need to help him? It is useless to deny or disregard the client's reality. Careful exploration, understanding and acceptance of the way things appear from the client's viewpoint are essential in creating helping relationships. The suggestion that alternative realities exist is more likely to be considered by the client who feels he has been understood. It is not unusual to find that incontinence is strongly denied by people whose world is crumbling around them because of it. No real start can be made in tackling the incontinence constructively until some acknowledgement of it as a reality is gained. This can require slow, patient work, in which the relationship forged between client and worker can be the chief means of overcoming the need for denial.

A substantial part of the problem solving process in social work practice can be termed 'manipulation of the environment'. Having established his goals, the client may see the need to alter some aspects of his environment that have a bearing on his problem. Social workers aim to ensure that clients themselves effect these helpful changes and develop confidence in their ability to pursue their own interests successfully. The social worker's role is supportive and enabling, ensuring that the client has access to resources and is able to secure them. There are times, however, when the social worker needs to act as advocate on behalf of his client, and times when he needs to act for his client if frailty, for example, prevents the client from acting for himself.

As mentioned above social services department personnel in all settings are constantly engaged in 'manipulation of the environment'. The effort to resolve problems posed by incontinence frequently involves the necessity to re-arrange accommodation, transport and daily routines, to secure a better understanding of difficulties and needs amongst those with whom the client lives or works and above all to secure medical assessment, diagnosis, treatment and advice. Social work principles of working towards self-help and self-confidence are important for all social services department personnel in helping the incontinent person to regain his self-esteem, but the necessity to be a determined advocate is also an essential role which should be willingly undertaken. Perhaps the most important awareness is that 'manipulation of the environment' is likely to be a necessary and worthwhile activity in respect of the problem posed by incontinence. By adjusting or changing environmental features, incontinence can often be overcome.

Training

Social services departments still organise some services on the basis of client groups and specific needs. Residential and day care facilities usually tend to concentrate on a particular aspect of need. Field social workers and domiciliary helpers are more likely to be working generically. In considering the knowledge and skills required by personnel working with incontinent clients, social services departments have a wide range of training and staff development needs to meet. Comparatively few members of staff in the many settings involved, will have any helpful or appropriate training in relation to the cause and effect of incontinence, its successful management or reversal. In relation to a condition in which physical and emotional factors can have a subtle interrelationship, it is obviously necessary for social services departments to seek the involvement of health service colleagues in training programmes. Staff (including foster parents) who are providing help with the physical needs of incontinent clients will need to gain confidence in methods of helping that are particularly suited to the setting in which the incontinent client requires help. Methods that are well suited to hospital-based management or even home nursing, might not be appropriate in a residential home or adult training centre for example.

It is essential that social services department personnel understand the origins of their clients' problems relating to incontinence and yet this is frequently not the case. Perhaps the guiding principle which training programmes should endeavour to convey is that incontinence should not be accepted as a feature of life unless it has been thoroughly investigated and the cause established. If treatment is recommended it should be pursued. If no treatment is thought appropriate, advice should be sought as to the best method of management, bearing in mind the need to maintain the client's dignity and self-esteem.

There are perhaps three main areas which social services department personnel could be helped to explore through training programmes. They would have differing degrees of significance depending on the setting and client group.

1. The Failure to Achieve Continence. Consideration of the very varied causes of failure to achieve continence would clarify the problems of clients, both children and adults, whose sphincter control has not developed as a result of congenital physical and/or mental handicap or because of severe emotional maladjustment (e.g. autism). Methods of management geared to particular needs could be demonstrated. All social services department personnel who provide support to congenitally handicapped clients and their families, would be better equipped for their task, if this clear background information were available.

2. Loss of continence as a Result of Trauma. Injury and disease can result in loss of the capacity for sphincter control at any stage in life. There is some possibility of social services department personnel in all settings encountering clients who have this adjustment to make. Once again, it is essential that training programmes emphasise the need to understand the causes of the incontinence in each case and whether there is any possibility that partial control can be regained and if so, how. The particular adjustments that have to be made will vary infinitely and social services department staff through training need some understanding of the stresses that the problem creates for children and young people, adults and the very old. The processes of adjustment, both practical and emotional, need to be understood also. The reactions of those most closely involved with the client need consideration since the successful adjustment of relatives and friends to the changed circumstances is likely to be a determining factor in successful management of them. Many relatives are not adequately helped and supported at this stage and subsequent breakdown of goodwill often relates to this initial neglect. Beyond adjustment the aim should be to ensure that the client regains his sense of purpose in life and, if at all possible, is enabled to live with little real impediment from his residual disabilities. Training programmes can ensure that social services department staff gain awareness of the helping process in rehabilitation and specific information about aids and appliances which enable incontinence to be managed with a minimum of fuss.

3. Loss of Continence as a Result of a Combination of Factors in Old Age. Incontinence and old age are readily seen as synonymous. A pattern is established and perhaps successfully concealed for a time. When brought to light, it is still very likely that no effort will be made to find out why the person is incontinent, when, and in what circumstances it began. There is likely to be no clear picture of what is happening. Social workers, occupational therapists, home-helps, residential staff, and day centre staff can all become caught up in the unclear yet problematical circumstances, together with colleagues in the primary health care team. Crisis and breakdown in the elderly person's life frequently centre upon his incontinence and yet reasons for incontinence are not established. Joint training programmes with health service personnel would have particular value in encouraging more understanding of what can be done.

There is a need to unravel the events and influences that lead towards incontinence in old age. Acute and chronic ill-health, disabling diseases and mobility problems play their part. Stressful events such as bereavement and any sudden unwelcome changes which threaten security and well-being, are of great significance. Environmental factors which effectively reduce ease of access to lavatories are obviously determining factors but are sometimes extremely difficult to recognise as such by those who are familiar with them. Patterns such as alcoholism and mild, chronic depression (either acknowleged or hidden) can reduce the motivation that is needed to maintain continence. The real difficulty can be that a number of causative factors are at work together and the skill lies in determining whether any of them is of greater significance than the others, or whether it is the combination of all the factors that must be dealt with.

The use of case material is a necessary part of the training programme in order to build up awareness of how events combine to produce the established pattern of incontinence, and to illustrate the various ways of intervening. It is also important that methods whereby support and encouragement are offered to old people coping with multiple handicaps are considered. The effort which has to be made in order to overcome problems such as incontinence or to achieve an agreeable life-style despite them is very great. So many other challenges and deprivations have to be met in old age. Social services department personnel require the ability to assess strengths and vulnerabilities in their elderly clients and devise the strategies that will maximise the former whilst reducing stress in the more vulnerable areas. Finally, training programmes should aim to strengthen awareness of the available resources, and how they can be secured, both from within and from without social services departments. The many skills that are available in all fields, both statutory and voluntary, should be clarified and the way in which they can be deployed should be understood. For example, the precise nature of the help that the occupational therapist can offer with regard to assessment, aids to daily living and adaptation of housing should be known. The physiotherapist's ability, in some cases, to teach exercises for pelvic muscles, which can gradually reduce the incidence of stress incontinence, should be known.

In examining the diversity of skills that can be called upon in the effort to combat incontinence, social services department personnel can be helped to recognise their part in a multidisciplinary team effort. The importance of effective working relationships can be considered in relation to:

(1) exposing the problem and the needs;
(2) proper assessment;
(3) implementing treatment plans; and
(4) supporting the client, his family and others.

In the daily welter of work it is perhaps difficult for staff, in their varied activities, to feel part of a team effort. It is not as though, for example, there is the regular opportunity for care assistant, general practitioner, occupational therapist and social worker to meet and plan how best to help Mrs Brown (who might live in the old people's home), to overcome the problem of incontinence. Nevertheless, the care assistant *must* feel confident that her regular contact with Mrs Brown and her recorded observations of the daily pattern of Mrs Brown's bladder function, are essential in 'exposing the problem and the need'. Unless this first step is taken, those with special skill and knowledge will not be brought into the picture. Proper assessment of the problem and all that then follows, hinges on the ability of those working most closely with the client, to recognise what is happening and make it known. The ability and confidence can be developed through appropriate training. The implementation of treatment plans is also likely to depend on the 'front line' helpers: families, home-helps, family helpers, care assistants, foster parents, etc. They need to feel clear about the aims of the treatment plan, how to undertake it, and who will be supporting them. A sense of teamwork can then develop, despite the lack of a true team structure.

The Elderly Person in Residential Care

For months now we have had trouble with him urinating on the bedroom floor and in the wash-bowl. When the night staff have checked the urine bottle that he has in his room, he has emptied it either through the window or down the wash-bowl.

The staff do not have the chance to empty the bottle, although they have tried, by checking every half-hour, because he empties it as soon as he has used it.

He has been seen urinating in the wash-bowl and denied it at the time and he has had as many as three urine bottles at the same time, which he has taken himself, but these have been hidden in his wardrobe.

We had to move him from one double room which he was sharing, because he was using the other resident's hand towel as well as his own, to urinate into. Also with emptying the urine bottle into, and urinating into, the wash-bowl, the tiles were stained and came up from the floor, even though they were washed every time they were found wet. They were scrubbed, dried and re-set again.

We have tried every conceivable method of treatment, but to no avail. He is at present in a double room on his own, and I have to admit another man into the room. This is very worrying, due to the problems another man had when sharing the room, and his behaviour, if anything, is worse now.

All his clothes have to be kept away from him, to keep them clean, and his towel has to be put outside his room at night.

He is not incontinent during the day but does wet the toilet floor and goes to his bedroom and urinates in a towel. He is able to do the crossword in the *Daily Mail* every day, but he does take some items such as cushions and cardigans which belong to the ladies. He is not on any medication at night to cause 'confusion'.

This report from a puzzled head of a home for elderly people illustrates the issues and concerns regularly arising around the occurrence of incontinence. As suggested earlier, incontinence in elderly people is likely to have a complex aetiology and the progress towards successful management is likely to be equally complex. It can be difficult to pinpoint the exact context in which incontinence began. The example given states 'for months now . . .', so it was not always so; but what was happening at the time it began, or just before it began? Will anyone be able to remember? It might be extremely important that this is recalled.

Adequate recording of the events in elderly people's lives is necessary in a group setting such as a residential home. Significant events, experiences and reactions can so quickly be forgotten. Adequate recording implies adequate staff time and skill and proper deployment. Where staff are deployed in task-centred rather than client-centred activity, the opportunity to develop effective relationships with people in residential care will be greatly diminished. Without these relationships, it will be difficult to ensure recognition of the significant day-to-day experiences of each person in the group. The example above shows that staff have given a lot of time to observing what is going on. (They have never found the urine bottle full, always empty, 'through window, down wash-bowl'. Did he ever use it?) The nature of the relationships and the quality of the communication with this man are not clear however. He denied urinating in his wash-bowl so it seems likely that he was accused of doing so. Urine bottles are 'hidden' rather than 'kept'. Are there constructive relationships and helpful communication, or are things cool and strained? Has he been encouraged to participate fully in all the steps that have been taken or have his clothes been removed and his room changed without full discussion and agreement with him? Is the unspoken communciation likely to be as follows? 'You have dirty habits which you are deliberately using to make life difficult for us and everyone else here. We don't like your dirty habits, they mess up our home. If you carry on like this you won't be able to stay here. We've done all we can.'

Where staff activity in residential homes is not constructively client-centred at all times, issues such as cleanliness and hygiene, both of the building and its inmates can take on disproportionate importance. Work then, is about the rota of staff duties, tasks and routines, rather than about thoughtful response to needs (both tangible and intangible) of the elderly people. Non-verbal messages are usually very clear to those to whom they are directed. Incontinence can be a powerful reaction in a situation in which personal needs are ignored, denied or rejected. Within residential homes for elderly people, life-style based on large groups and task-centred staff routines can create the likelihood that personal needs will not be met adequately. With sound relationships it is possible to counsel and advise when there are difficulties. Without sound relationships there is no basis for working through complex problems. In homes for elderly people staff need the time and the ability to establish relationships with clients and to counsel them. 'Antisocial' behaviour cannot be resolved to order or by 'treatment', but it might well yield to empathy and concern.

Within homes for the elderly can be found a high level of unassessed incontinence. There are brain-damaged but active people urinating and defecating in the 'wrong' places and handling or eating faeces. There are those who appear to lack all motivation and are perhaps persistently mildly depressed. Others might well be communicating their feelings by means of incontinence. (One elderly man exhibiting faecal incontinence, said following a period of constructive counselling in which a number of issues were resolved, 'I don't need to be dirty any more, it's served its purpose'.) Some might have a way of coping that merits the tag 'dirty habits'. There are those with catheters, and those who deny any question of incontinence but who carefully make parcels and leave them in other people's lockers. There are those with ill-health, organic problems, and disabilities affecting mobility. It is a great tribute to residential staff that they manage as well as they do with little in the way of help and support from the health service and often without adequate information and equipment.

Demands and expectations concerning the management of incontinent elderly people in residential homes have grown considerably during the last decade. The most recent Ministry of Health guidelines (MOH circular 10/65) have indicated that people with 'intractable' incontinence and other disabilities should only be admitted to residential homes if the condition has been fully assessed and treated. If treatment cannot reverse the condition, a method of management should have been put into effect. There is however, a growing expectation that incontinence, at the point of admission, will be acceptable despite lack of assessment, treatment or a sound method of management.

At best, 'method of management' is likely to be an indwelling catheter, especially if the new resident has been admitted from hospital.

Apart from the fact that a catheter is often demoralising to the person who is trying to find his place in a strange group environment which is to be his new home, it is not always easy to ensure the necessary help with the management of the catheter from the primary health care team.

Much of the frustration and concern experienced by residental staff in connection with incontinence relates to the conflict that arises when trying to provide a service which they feel to be outside the remit of Part III accommodation as reflected in present staffing levels, conditions of service, training, knowledge and skills. It might be a very different picture if assessment, diagnosis, treatment and support with management of incontinence and other health problems were readily and adequately available from the health service. It can be difficult to get the elderly person referred to the geriatrician or other appropriate specialist in the first place.

The lack of assessment and treatment reflects two main difficulties. The first is the attitude that accepts incontinence as a feature of old age, so that 'nothing can be done', and there is 'no point' in referral for specialist help. The second is the shortage of skilled personnel and other resources in the health service in relation to the rapidly-growing numbers of elderly people needing help. Priorities are drawn up and services are 'rationed'. People needing careful investigation can be excluded from acute hospital beds by virtue of the fact that they are aged over 65. There might be the offer of two weeks 'assessment' in a 'holiday' bed in a geriatric unit. 'Turnover' and 'through-put' are perhaps more pressing than successful amelioration of the diagnosed condition. Homes for the elderly are viewed by many in the health service as annexes to the geriatric unit and the psychiatric ward. In some areas the policy whereby psychiatric provision has been pared away, results in mentally ill old people being admitted to or contained in Part III homes.

In this climate, there is real conflict for residential staff who are genuinely concerned to improve the quality of the experience of elderly people in care and who wish to respond to the challenge spelt out in reports such as that of the Personal Social Services Council, 'Residential Care Reviewed'. A residential home overwhelmed by the effort to keep old people fed, clean, dry, and regularly toileted has little capacity to offer more. The sheer bulk of foul linen in some homes preoccupies the thoughts and efforts of the staff team. Budget priority is given to securing a *second* large-capacity foul-linen washing machine . . .

The reluctance to admit to residential care those elderly people known to be already incontinent is balanced all too often by the resignation with which it is accepted that the new resident *becomes* incontinent soon after admission. Admission to residential care is a crisis in the life of the elderly person and even where there has been good preparation and careful introduction, trauma cannot be eliminated. Seen through the eyes of the client, the period preceding admission is likely to have been stressful. A decision had to be made and this must have involved the acknowledgement of the breakdown of a familiar pattern of coping. The past events of life have probably been mulled over and old pleasures and pains recalled. Relationships have been scrutinised; is the account in credit or showing a heavy loss through bereavement and other departures? Perhaps it has been necessary to go through treasured possessions which are symbols of happier days. They have to be given up. Privacy, a further treasure, of growing value in recent years, will be lost. Behind it all is a nagging sense of failure. Then there are the uncertainities:

> Will I like it? Will 'they' like me? Will I be able to manage well enough, find my way, get help if I need it, in the strange surroundings? What about the nights, I sleep so badly and I have to share . . . I can't eat a lot of things, will I manage?

Prior to admission, field social workers must be able to respond to these concerns and prepare both client and residential staff adequately. On admission, so much will depend on how staff help to pave the way. The attitudes and sensitivity they convey will either create the basis for trust and confidence or add to the stress of the initial experience. Good admission procedure will ensure that all available necessary information about the client's needs has been carefully considered and shared with staff, that time is set aside to discuss special needs and difficulties thoroughly and to show the layout of the home, pointing out the essential facilities carefully. The daily routines will be described and someone appointed to be friend and guide during the early days. Introductions will be made properly and not left to chance. Faulty admission procedure or lack of sensitivity on the part of staff can heighten the effect of the stress and uncertainty that the decisions leading up to admission have created, and the newly admitted person is very vulnerable. Confusion, sudden physical deterioration and incontinence have been known to develop within a short period after admission. Devastating to the elderly person, this sequence of events is demoralising to staff whose already limited resources are further burdened by the effort to help overcome the breakdown.

Time, sound procedures, skill, confidence and sensitivity are some of the basic needs of residential staff who are expected to provide a good service to vulnerable old people. In the effort to prevent or overcome problems such as incontinence in residential homes however, other things can be of equal importance.

1. Life Style

Homes for the elderly have traditionally offered care on a fairly indiscriminate basis (i.e. everyone is helped with bathing whether necessary or otherwise; everyone's clothes are laundered for them; everyone's tea is served to them etc.). Life is spent as one of a number in a large group with no particular role to fulfil (other than to be a recipient of 'care'), or demands to meet. There is little privacy, since bedrooms are frequently multi-bedded and this tends to influence the way in which bathing and toiletting routines are managed as well.

In recent years, the undermining effects of this life-style have been recognised. Some homes have been designed and built to create the opportunity for people to live in small groups of eight or so, each with their own bedroom; some existing homes have adapted the building to make re-organisation from large to small group-living a possibility. The essential feature of this change is that the group of elderly people have access to their own living area comprising a small, domestic-type kitchen and a lounge/dining room. Ordinary day-to-day tasks such as preparing and serving meals and washing up afterwards can be undertaken by the group, helping one another. Housework in the group's living area (or 'flat') is undertaken by group members. Decisions about everyday routines as well as special events (e.g. how a birthday will be celebrated), are made by the group members. There is the need for interaction and sharing. The effort must be made to resolve problems (especially those of interpersonal relationships), and make decisions.

Frail and heavily-handicapped people, those with problems relating to atherosclerotic changes etc., are demonstrating their ability to cope with this life-style and to derive real satisfaction from it. Amongst the many benefits that appear to stem from this way of life are greater concern about personal standards, appearance and dress etc., less preoccupation with food itself as the highlight to the day and more real concern for the well-being of others in the group. Staff have found that old people themselves try to ensure that the lavatories are used with consideration for 'the person who uses it next', and that they get to the lavatory in good time to keep themselves dry. Much less food seems to be eaten compared with the piled plates in traditional-style homes. The sick or dying resident is comforted and watched over. The part that staff play in the home is supportive and facilitating. Assessment of the need rather than the pursuit of regular care routines is uppermost.

The dynamic atmosphere generated by this life-style throws into relief the apathy and withdrawal that is still sometimes to be found in the traditional-style home, where work is task-centred and relates to a large group. Incontinence is something for staff to manage rather than a personal difficulty that the elderly person is helped to overcome. Special areas in the home are sometimes set aside as 'wet wings' in order to make it possible for hard-pressed staff to manage. Inmates of the 'wet wings' are termed the 'babies' and this pseudonym no doubt makes it easier for staff to bear the unpleasant tasks they undertake. A high proportion of staff time is given to the 'babies'. Those who are not incontinent receive proportionately less time as a result. But when other rewarding relationships are few or non-existent, how many continent old people start to wet themselves as a means to securing personal attention from staff? The significance of relationships and personal recognition was made clear in the incident when an active old lady, who was being 'habit trained' by means of regular supervised trips to the lavatory, presented herself to the care assistant and told her 'it's time for me to go now.'

Many social services departments are giving thought to the effects of life-style in homes for the elderly. Dramatic improvement in resident and staff morale can result from a well-organised approach to change.

2. Design and Layout

The design features that enable the small group life-style in homes for the elderly are also those most likely to minimise the incontinence which results from inaccessible lavatories. People with urge incontinence and mobility problems must be within easy reach of lavatories if they are to manage. The living areas for small groups are relatively compact which makes things easier. Some of the older purpose-built homes, as well as the adapted homes, present formidable distances for people to walk. Fire regulations have resulted in the introduction of heavy fire doors at regular intervals along corridors. Some incontinence occurs simply because lavatories are situated on the far side of the fire door which the elderly person, perhaps using a walking-aid, cannot open in time.

There must be an adequate number of lavatories. Rhythms being what they are, a high proportion of people need to use the lavatory around the same time as others each day. Frail old people cannot wait and queue in quite the same way as younger people. In one old adapted house there was one lavatory, and another within a bathroom, to be shared by 22 people. The congestion in the early morning was such that a number of residents became severely constipated because they could not gain access to the lavatory when they needed to open their bowels. Constipation can lead to impaction and to 'overflow' diarrhoea, so the fact that the drainage system in this house could not support any more lavatories created a very serious design limitation with regard to the prevention of incontinence.

The Department of Health and Social Security Building Notes for homes for the elderly give guidance to local authorities on all essential features of design, layout and facilities, including provision of lavatories. Perhaps in the current economic climate it will not be possible for local authorities to add to the number of new residential homes. In upgrading existing homes however, one of the priorities is to create more toilet provision. If new homes are to be built, consideration should be given to providing bedrooms with integral lavatory and hand washbasin. This would go a long way to reducing the incidence of incontinence and also the indignity and inconvenience arising from the use of commodes.

3. Admission Policies

Local authority homes for the elderly have a statutory duty to fulfil, which is to provide 'accommodation for those in need of care and attention not otherwise available'. Homes are thus frequently seen as able to absorb whoever has the greatest need for the service at the point when the vacancy arises. In addition to the expectation that homes will respond to need on demand, there is a further implicit and often explicit expectation, that homes will ensure a good experience for the new resident. The resident is expected to be 'happier' as a result of entering the home.

There is much evidence, however, to suggest that these expectations are not necessarily compatible. Life in a group is a dynamic, changing experience offering different opportunities and posing different limitations as time goes by. It is not static and unvarying, however much to an outsider this might seem to be the case. Conflicting needs within the group create stresses, tensions and even crises, which the staff may or may not have the capacity to deal with at the time. Staff come and go, are sick, and are at varying stages in their own resourcefulness and skill. The building which houses the home, may be disrupted by repairs, adaptations, redecoration etc. When a vacancy occurs in the home, it is important for the well-being of the new resident, the existing residents and the staff, that the capacity of the home to meet additional needs is matched as nearly as possible with the needs of the new resident. In a home where, for example, residents and staff are all suffering the stress created by a high proportion of incontinent people, and where the laundry facilities are due for re-organisation next week, it can be disastrous to admit another incontinent person whose continence is suspect, however great this need may be. Residential staff need help and support in trying to achieve reasonable, balanced work loads. In this way they will retain the capacity to provide care and attention and will be more likely to enable residents to find life in a group a worthwhile and enabling experience, in which they can overcome their difficulties.

4. Teamwork

Residential staff cannot be expected to manage the complex combination of personal need that is embodied in a large group of elderly people, without help. Physical and mental health problems, including incontinence, are extensive in this group of clients. First, field social workers who are introducing the elderly person to residential care need to provide adequate accurate information and must obtain from the general practitioner a comprehensive report in relation to physical and mental health. Medical certificates prior to admission are often only sketchily completed. Information concerning medication is not always comparable with the recently-prescribed medicines that the new resident brings to the home. Information concerning bowel and bladder function is most essential together with the reasons for any difficulties, the treatment that has been tried, etc.

Then, the residential staff need support from the general practitioner if there are significant health problems which do not yield to the treatment he prescribes. Referral for specialist medical advice where necessary should be pursued, on humane grounds primarily, but also because untreated health problems can ultimately outstrip the staff's capacity to cope. Incontinence is one of the conditions which is unlikely to be referred for specialist medical advice – it should be.

Some residential homes have a medical officer in addition to the general practitioners who attend individual residents. The functions of the medical officer have recently been restated by the Department of Health and Social Security in 'A Memorandum of Guidance on Arrangements for Health Care, Residential Homes for the Elderly' (Paragraphs 35-9). It is a role which can be supportive to residential staff over matters such as incontinence, where information and advice concerning appropriate resources and equipment are needed. A medical officer can also presumably help residential staff by, for example, stating the case to management for additional lavatories. It is less clear as to whether the medical officer can act as advocate at times when a general practitioner is not willing to refer his incontinent patient for specialist advice or when the geriatrician is pressing the home to re-accept from hospital a former resident who remains incontinent or who has been 'treated' by means of an indwelling catheter. Residential staff are often in need of help in these circumstances.

Where the geriatrician and the psychiatrist have good working relationships with residential staff and are willing to give advice in respect of elderly people who have been their patients, difficulties are likely to be managed with greater success. As has been described earlier, assessment, diagnosis, and treatment or effective management of incontinence require close co-operation between everyone concerned. Treatment and management plans must relate realistically to the environment in which the person lives.

Thus an elderly lady was admitted to a residential home from the psychiatric unit. Although not incontinent she was obviously totally pre-occupied with the imminence of this catastrophe. She could not rest a minute and spent the day trekking to and from the lavatory, saying to anyone who needed her attention 'Sorry, can't stop, my boilers are bursting.' Her distress and restlessness concerned the staff and other residents but neither her doctor nor the psychiatrist attached much importance to it. It took real determination on the part of the staff to convey successfully the wretchedness of the old lady's condition and her inability to get anything out of life in the home. The psychiatrist's suggestion that a nominal amount of a familiar drug might reduce the agitation proved dramatically accurate. Almost overnight the preoccupation with her bladder disappeared and she became able to relate to her surroundings more naturally.

A further essential member of the team effort in residential homes is the community nurse. Residential staff are not expected to be nurses even if they possess nursing qualifications. Where nursing procedures are to be undertaken the community nurse should be responsible for them in association with residential staff. Management of incontinence by means of a catheter should always be supported by the community nurse. In some areas there are not enough nurses to meet all the demands for their services and local priorities may result in old people in residential homes being deprived of this service. In view of the high concentration of need in residential homes, decisions such as these should be carefully reconsidered.

Sheltered Housing

Some elderly people in sheltered housing and warden-attended schemes are supported by social services department personnel such as social workers, therapists and home-helps, etc. Problems amongst these tenants intensify as they become older. The limited role of the warden is not adequate to deal with the level of frailty and handicap that is emerging. Incontinence is a growing feature of the difficulties the wardens and home-helps strive to manage. Tenants and their families look to the wardens and expect them to be able to cope with responsibilities which are beyond their brief. Consideration needs to be given by health and social services to ways of augmenting support to the housing schemes. Developments such as that devised in Southampton between the housing department, health and social services and put into practice at Kinloss Court, will perhaps prove to be a pattern for the future.

Implications for Management

Social services departments have many major pressing demands on their resources. What likelihood is there that any attention, let alone priority, will be given by those who make policy decisions to a relatively hidden affliction such as incontinence? Although hidden, it is, as Dorothy Mandelstam has made clear 'a very common complaint'[1] with the possibility of two million sufferers in Britain. Where the condition is not adequately ameliorated, there exists the likelihood of crisis and breakdown about which something has to be done. Social services department personnel, as has been shown, are frequently the people called upon to act. Resources are being used and these are costly. Attention is merited therefore and the strategy should be:

(1) to devise clear policies in relation to the areas of the social services department's involvement with incontinence, which are designed to ensure a consistent, integrated approach; joint

planning with health service colleagues should be undertaken in respect of policies and resources;

(2) to develop training programmes appropriate to the varied roles and responsibilities of social services department personnel;

(3) to ensure adequate basic facilities and resources with which to promote continence and facilitate the management of incontinence; and

(4) to use the opportunities open to social services departments in order to negotiate a proper understanding of incontinence in other helping agencies and in the community generally.

Note

1. Mandelstam, D. (1977), *Incontinence* (Heinemann, London).

14 THE PREVALENCE AND HEALTH SERVICE IMPLICATIONS OF INCONTINENCE

Thelma M. Thomas

Urinary incontinence is a common symptom which can affect people of all ages. It is a manifestation of a variety of different pathological processes and occurs in association with a number of different diagnoses. In addition it can vary in severity both in terms of quantity and frequency of leakage, and in terms of the degree of handicap that has been incurred.[1-12]

Faecal incontinence is less common than urinary incontinence and as an isolated symptom should persist only rarely, almost all cases being treatable. On the other hand, persisting double incontinence is not uncommon particularly in special groups such as the mentally handicapped or confused elderly.[11-13]

When dealing with such a protean symptom there are a number of questions to be answered before the problem as seen in hospital or general practice can be put into its real perspective in terms of its prevalence and implications in the population as a whole.

Firstly, a definition of the symptom is needed so that studies from different sources can be compared. Ideally this definition should be an objective one. However, in the absence of a quick, low cost, highly sensitive test a subjective definition must suffice for a community-based study. In addition to such a definition, there needs to be an assessment of the effects of the symptom on the sufferer and/or carers as what is a major impediment to one may be a minor inconvenience to another. This variation in symptom perception may be only partly influenced by associated handicaps such as mobility problems. It is necessary to identify these associated problems, and also to examine in detail services and medical help available for, and in use by, the incontinent population.

Finally, there needs to be an estimate of the number of incontinent people who are not receiving any help with an assessment of the severity of their symptomatology and of the extent to which extra medical and other help might be beneficial and acceptable.

It was to answer some of these questions that the Medical Research Council's study of the prevalence and health and social service implications of incontinence was initiated in 1976.[14-18] The main studies were carried out in two London health districts; all residents aged five years and over were included. Residents from the districts living in institutions outside the study area were also included. Additional studies were carried out in two other areas. The definition of incontinence used throughout the study was involuntary excretion or leakage of urine and/or faeces in inappropriate places or at inappropriate times and producing two or more 'accidents' a month or continuous leakage of urine. Patients with long-term catheters and urinary diversions were included.

Recognised Incontinence

In order to identify incontinent patients in touch with health and social service agencies in Brent and Harrow contact was made with representatives from each of the agencies shown in Table 14.1. They were asked to notify, for a year, all patients who were incontinent according to the survey definition. Each patient's age, sex, address and the type of incontinence − urinary, faecal or both − were recorded.

Table 14.1: Health and Social Service Sources

Geriatric wards − acute, medium and long-stay
Psychiatric wards − acute and long-stay
Unit for younger chronic sick
Hospital for mentally handicapped
Old people's homes
Day centres
Special schools
District nurses, health visitors
Laundry service, pad service
Multiple Sclerosis Society, Association for Spina Bifida

Patients who were living at home or who were identified while in an acute geriatric ward were interviewed by a nurse from the survey team using a structured questionnaire about the type and severity of incontinence, associated disabilities, management and services received.

A total of 2,005 incontinent patients aged 15 and over were identified, of whom 656 (33 per cent) were doubly incontinent and 55 (3 per cent) incontinent of faeces alone. The estimated total study population aged 15 or over was 359,000. The prevalence estimates derived from these figures are shown in Table 14.2. In addition 119 handicapped children with urinary and/or faecal incontinence were identified.

Table 14.2: Prevalence of Recognised Incontinence per 1,000 Population

| | At Home | | In Institution | |
	Urinary incontinence (including double)	Faecal incontinence (including double)	Urinary incontinence (including double)	Faecal incontinence (including double)
15-64 Male	0.5	0.2	0.5	0.3
Female	1.1	0.2	0.7	0.3
65 + Male	8.0	2.0	6.0	3.1
Female	10.4	2.2	14.6	6.9

A greater proportion of those in long-stay institutions were doubly incontinent than of those living at home (Table 14.3).

Table 14.3: Type of Incontinence (excluding faecal)

			Urinary (%)	Double (%)	Total (100%)
Males	15-64	At home	47 (67)	23 (33)	70
		Institution	31 (44)	40 (56)	71
	65 +	At home	183 (78)	50 (22)	233
		Institution	93 (53	81 (47)	174
Females	15-64	At home	140 (86)	22 (14)	162
		Institution	57 (50)	57 (50)	114
	65 +	At home	385 (82)	83 (18)	468
		Institution	358 (54)	300 (46)	658
Total			1294 (66)	656 (34)	1950

Of the 933 adults who were incontinent of urine (or doubly incontinent) and living at home, 671 (72 per cent) were interviewed (164 aged 15 to 64 and 507 aged 65 and over). Also interviewed were the parents of 100 (84 per cent) of the handicapped children.

Of the adult referrals 95 per cent were followed up for a year. During that time 2 per cent moved out of the area; 37 per cent of the elderly and 10 per cent of those under 65 died; 5 per cent ceased to be incontinent.

The Elderly at Home Aged 65 and Over

About 80 per cent of the elderly interviewed were able to answer for themselves, although a few (9 per cent) did not admit that they were incontinent. Otherwise information was obtained from carers. One-fifth of the men and one-third of the women lived alone at the time of the first interview. Thirty-five per cent of the total were fully mobile or limited only by slowness or limping while 42 per cent used aids to move around and 23 per cent were chair- or bed-bound. Sixty per cent had been incontinent for longer than a year. Wetting occurred at least once every 24 hours in 68 per cent. It occurred by day and by night in 58 per cent; by day only in 25 per cent and by night only in 17 per cent.

In the majority (about 90 per cent) of cases it was possible to ascribe medical diagnoses which could have been causative of or contributory to the incontinence. For example:

One-fifth were hemiplegic
27 per cent of the women but only 38 per cent of the men had
  some form of disabling arthritis
about 10 per cent showed evidence of dementia
6 per cent were diabetic
6 per cent had Parkinson's disease
Over half had two or more relevant diagnoses.

All current medications were noted with especial reference to groups of drugs of possible relevance to the management of incontinence. These were:

Diuretics taken by 37 per cent
Digoxin taken by 12 per cent
Sedatives and tranquillisers taken by 17 per cent
Hypnotics taken by 28 per cent
Constipating mixtures taken by 1 per cent
Laxatives taken by 17 per cent
Drugs for urinary incontinence taken by 4 per cent
One-third were taking drugs from two or more of these groups.

Permanent indwelling urethral catheters were being used by 27 (17 per cent) of the men and 21 (6 per cent) of the women while a further seven men (4 per cent) had fixed appliances or condoms. Three women had ileal conduits.

A district nurse was visiting 30 per cent of the elderly for reasons specifically to do with bladder or bowel care. Over two-thirds were receiving pads via the local pad service. A delivery system operated in one of the districts where there was also a collection service, although this was not very popular because of the distinctive red bags which were provided. In the other district pads had to be collected from a clinic or were delivered by the community nurse. A number of problems were identified in both districts which were subsequently examined and the service adjusted. For example, in one district the standard pads being provided to patients or carers who called to collect them were polythene backed and not designed for use in the plastic pants provided. They also needed cutting which was very difficult for a number of the elderly or disabled. In this district too, at this time, marsupial Kanga pants were available but only at the discretion of the community nurse for patients being visited by the nurses. The ambulant incontinent patients for whom they were designed might, therefore, not have been able to obtain them. Ideally, all new incontinent patients should be assessed at the outset by a community nurse and this was recommenced soon after these surveys took place.

Where the delivery system was used it was proving difficult to tailor the service to adjust for variations in need. About one in seven people said they were receiving too many pads while an almost identical number said they were receiving too few. The service was very dependent on the interest and enthusiasm of the drivers employed — an interested driver relayed messages and checked that deliveries were received successfully. However, when the driver did not fulfil this function communications were often poor because recipients of the service did not have a single reliable phone number they could contact to query their supply. A problem in both districts was that of ensuring that both the incontinent people or their carers and the health care professionals involved were fully conversant with the supplies available.

Because incontinence supplies are bulky, storage can be a problem and thus careful timing of orders and reliable delivery from stockists is essential if adequate supplies are to be maintained for collection or delivery. A greater understanding of the nature of the problem by supplies officers, clinic clerks or others involved in the service should help towards ensuring a caring service which is efficient and effective.

Nearly 60 per cent of the elderly using pads disposed of them in the dustbin, 16 per cent used a collection service, 6 per cent burnt them indoors and 11 per cent outdoors. A small proportion (7 per cent) flushed them away.

Although 71 per cent of those interviewed had some extra laundry because of their incontinence, only 8 per cent were using the local laundry service. Use of a laundry service is often limited because of the need to have a lot of sheets (though this was obviated in one district with the introduction of a supply of bed linen). Only 12 per cent of the men and 30 per cent of the women were doing their own laundry but it was being done by a resident relative or friend for a further 68 per cent of elderly men and 42 per cent of the elderly women. Home washing machines were used by 35 per cent.

Considerable help was being given by family and friends. Over two-thirds of the group were receiving some regular assistance from resident or visiting family or friends. In over 50 per cent of cases this included help specifically to do with bladder or bowel management. Nearly 40 per cent of the elderly were receiving help daily and a further 40 per cent were being helped by day and by night.

Everyone able to answer for themselves was asked what was the worst problem they had in managing their daily life. Only 5 per cent said that the management of their incontinence was their worst problem, while 24 per cent said it was their limited mobility. Similarly in answer to a question about the worst aspect of managing their incontinence 38 per cent replied that their limited mobility was the worst factor.

Patients or their carers were shown a list of services and asked whether they felt any would be of help to them. One-quarter of those answering identified one or more which they felt might be of benefit. Of these nearly half had tried to contact the services but had not been successful in obtaining them.

Incontinent Adults (age range 15-64) Receiving Help at Home

The majority of this group suffered from a chronic disabling neurological condition — 53 (32 per cent) had multiple sclerosis, 17 (10 per cent) were hemiplegic. A further 19 (12 per cent) were mentally handicapped.

A small proportion (2 per cent of men and 12 per cent of women) lived alone. Only 30 per cent of the men but nearly 60 per cent of the women could walk without the use of aids. Over 90 per cent had been incontinent for longer than a year. Wetting occurred at least once every 24 hours in 58 per cent. It occurred by day and by night in 49 per cent, by day only in 36 per cent and by night only in 15 per cent.

A quarter of the group were being visited by a district nurse for reasons specifically to do with bladder or bowel care. Nearly 60 per cent were using pads provided locally. Only 27 per cent used the collection service; 41 per cent disposed of them in the dustbin; 6 per cent burnt them indoors and 3 per cent outdoors; 23 per cent flushed them away. Although 63 per cent had extra laundry because of their incontinence, only 3 per cent were using the local laundry service. Four per cent of the men and 47 per cent of the women were doing their own extra laundry. Home washing machines were used by 62 per cent.

Over two-thirds were receiving some regular assistance from resident or visiting family or friends. In 54 per cent of cases this was help specifically to do with bladder or bowel management. Nearly 26 per cent were receiving help daily and a further 51 per cent were being helped by day and by night.

Only 1 per cent said that the management of incontinence was their worst problem in managing their daily life while 31 per cent said that their limited mobility was their worst problem. When asked about the problems of managing incontinence 17 per cent cited limited mobility as the worst factor.

Thirty-four (20 per cent) of patients or carers said they felt that one or more of the listed services which they were not receiving would be of benefit to them and of those 16 (47 per cent) had tried to contact these services.

Handicapped Children

The majority of the one hundred severely handicapped children interviewed were attending day special schools in the two districts.

Thirty-two (58 per cent) of the 55 boys and 32 (71 per cent) of the 45 girls were doubly incontinent. Two-thirds (67 per cent) of the boys and almost half (49 per cent) of the girls were fully mobile or had only slightly impaired mobility while the remainder needed some form of mobility aid. Almost all (92 per cent) had been incontinent all their life. Wetting occurred at least daily in nearly two-thirds (63 per cent) and by day and by night in 61 per cent. One-fifth (21 per cent) were wet by night only.

In about two-thirds of the cases there had been no investigation or active management of the incontinence and it was apparent that the majority of the parents considered that wetting, and soiling too in those with double incontinence, was an inevitable accompaniment of other disabilities. One-third of the group were being toilet trained while a further six had had some toilet training in the past. Three of the children were using or had used a buzzer. Five had had catheters at some stage in the past. Seven had ileal conduits.

Incontinence caused extra laundry for three-quarters (77 per cent) of the families. Sixty-three of the children wore incontinence pads, which were delivered to their homes in 39 cases. Two-thirds of those using pads disposed of them in their dustbin; only seven used the local collection service.

In one of the districts detailed costings were carried out using 1977/8 costs.

In this district 89 per cent of the families had some extra costs, averaging £1.53 weekly. Of this sum, 95p was accounted for by washing costs. If the eight families with no extra costs are included, the figures are £1.36 and 92p respectively. A third of the families spent over £2, and two spent over £4 weekly.

Eleven families with extra washing costs had no washing machines and all but one would have found a machine useful. Of the 31 families

with washing problems but no tumble dryer, only 4 would have pre-
ferred not to have one — for reasons of space and running costs. Of the
80 per cent of families with extra laundry, half said they would use a
free service, although none knew it was available. Disinfectant, pants
and talcum powder or cream were the items most often purchased.
Disinfectant and nappies were the items, after washing, on which most
was spent by those who used them. There was no difference in overall
weekly costs by sex, though 23p per week more was spent on items
purchased for girls than boys, while 24p per week more was spent on
washing for boys. Costs tended to increase with age. Expenditure did
not vary with the degree of mobility of the child, nor with the ability
to speak. Costs were more than twice as high (£1.50) for the majority
where the child was faecally incontinent once a week or more or
incontinent of urine once a day or more (6 per cent with no costs)
than for the 15 per cent incontinent less often (72p) (35 per cent
with no costs).

On average families spent 10.3 hours per week on extra care for the
management of incontinence. One mother said she spent no extra
time, but another estimated she spent 42 hours a week on her severely
subnormal, doubly incontinent child. This family received no pads or
pants from the service which was, none the less, available and had
no washing machine or drier. There was no obvious association between
extra hours of care and age or mobility.

Eighty-eight per cent of the families were receiving some attendance
allowance. Those not receiving an allowance still spent as much on
incontinence management (£1.49 per week) as those who were but
their children required or received fewer hours of care. Seventeen per
cent of the families were receiving supplementary benefit but none had
received specific payments towards the management of incontinence.

*Incontinence in Acute and Long-stay Geriatric Wards and Other
Institutions*

All admissions to the acute geriatric wards in the two district hospitals
in the study area over the course of a year were monitored to determine
whether or not they were incontinent. In addition to those who ful-
filled the survey definition of incontinence, a record was kept of all
those who were incontinent because of acute or terminal illness. There
were 1774 admissions to the two hospitals of which 276 were re-
admissions. Of the 406 males admitted 119 (29 per cent) were regularly
incontinent of urine with a further 105 (26 per cent) having incontinence associated with an acute or terminal illness. Of the 1092 females,

274 (25 per cent) were regularly incontinent with a further 234 (21 per cent) having incontinence associated with an acute or terminal illness. The prevalence of incontinence in the longer-stay geriatric ward varied from 41 to 78 per cent. In the psychogeriatric wards 26 per cent of patients were incontinent, and in the long-stay hospital for the mentally handicapped 15 per cent were incontinent. Nineteen per cent of the residents in the local authority old age homes surveyed were incontinent. The same proportion (19 per cent) was found incontinent in the private nursing homes but fewer residents (11 per cent) in the private and voluntary old age homes were incontinent.

Unrecognised Incontinence

Unrecognised incontinence was studied by means of a postal questionnaire sent to all those aged five or more on the lists of 12 general practitioners — a total population of 22,430. The general practitioners sent letters to each of their patients aged 16 and over, explaining the study and asking them to complete the questionnaire. Parents were asked to fill in forms for children aged 5-16. Up to two reminders were sent at three-weekly intervals to those who did not reply initially. Those who did not want to take part were asked to return a blank form.

Questions on the symptoms of stress incontinence, urge incontinence and bed-wetting were asked, together with a question on wetting 'at any other times'. A question on faecal incontinence was also included. There were three categories of answers to each question — never, less than twice a month and twice or more a month. Patients were classified as 'never incontinent', 'occasionally incontinent' (less than twice a month), or 'regularly incontinent' (twice or more a month). Patients whose replies were ambiguous were classified as 'uncertain'. Women were asked how many babies they had had.

Replies were received from 18,084 (89 per cent) of the 20,398 patients who had not moved from the address shown on the practice record. An additional 390 (1.9 per cent) refused to take part. The response rate varied between the practices, the lowest being 80 per cent and the highest 95 per cent. The proportion of patients answering that they were incontinent varied little between practices and showed similar patterns with age.

Urinary Incontinence (including those doubly incontinent)

Tables 14.4 and 14.5 show the results by age for the men and women

Table 14.4: Community Prevalence of Urinary Incontinence in Men

Age (years)	Never incontinent (%)	Occasionally incontinent (%)	Regularly incontinent (%)	Uncertain (%)	Total (100%)
5 – 14	1367 (81)	184 (11)	116 (7)	17 (1)	1684
15 – 24	1267 (95)	28 (2)	19 (1)	14 (1)	1328
25 – 34	1146 (95)	34 (3)	10 (1)	20 (2)	1210
35 – 44	1161 (94)	31 (2)	18 (1)	28 (2)	1238
45 – 54	1096 (93)	43 (4)	19 (2)	17 (1)	1175
55 – 64	909 (89)	58 (6)	30 (3)	27 (3)	1024
65 – 74	637 (81)	66 (8)	48 (6)	39 (5)	790
75 – 84	206 (75)	26 (10)	22 (8)	19 (7)	273
85 +	27 (69)	1 (3)	6 (15)	5 (13)	39
Total	7816 (89)	471 (6)	288 (3)	186 (2)	8761

Table 14.5: Community Prevalence of Urinary Incontinence in Women

Age (years)	Never incontinent (%)	Occasionally incontinent (%)	Regularly incontinent (%)	Uncertain (%)	Total (100%)
5 – 14	1284 (82)	175 (11)	80 (5)	17 (1)	1556
15 – 24	1065 (82)	154 (12)	52 (4)	20 (2)	1291
25 – 34	949 (72)	263 (20)	72 (6)	31 (2)	1315
35 – 44	816 (67)	254 (21)	125 (10)	32 (3)	1227
45 – 54	771 (64)	264 (22)	142 (12)	29 (2)	1206
55 – 64	777 (67)	217 (19)	139 (12)	33 (3)	1166
65 – 74	733 (73)	146 (15)	88 (9)	34 (3)	1001
75 – 84	288 (63)	62 (14)	73 (16)	33 (7)	456
85 +	64 (61)	17 (16)	17 (16)	7 (7)	105
Total	6747 (72)	1552 (17)	788 (9)	236 (2)	9323

respectively. Urinary incontinence whether regular or occasional was more common in women than men at all ages except 5-14 years. Although low in men aged 15-64, the prevalence of regular urinary incontinence in men increased with increasing age after 35. The prevalence in women changed little between the ages of 35 and 64 but fell in those aged 65-74 and rose in those aged 75 and over.

Over two per cent of all replies received were recorded as uncertain because there was some difficulty in interpreting their responses. More of the elderly returned uncertain replies than did those aged 65 years or under. There was a slightly higher proportion of uncertain replies from the women than from the men.

A review of the forms returned which had been marked uncertain enabled some deductions to be made about the uncertain responses. It was estimated that up to half of these replies could have been from people with regular urinary incontinence. However, these were not included with the positives because of the doubt involved.

The results for the 5-14 age group were analysed for each one year group and these results are shown in Tables 14.6 and 14.7. Urinary incontinence was commonest in the youngest children. About 90 per cent of the incontinent boys aged 5-14 had nocturnal enuresis. However only 65 per cent of the incontinent girls were bed-wetters, most of the remainder complained of urge incontinence.

Figure 14.1 shows the prevalence of regular incontinence by ten-year age groups in women aged 15 and over, with the proportion of each age group reporting urge incontinence only, stress incontinence only and combined urge and stress incontinence. Women reporting urinary incontinence only at 'other times' in reply to the postal questionnaire are omitted. (These replies accounted for only 1.8 per cent of the total.) The lower prevalence in the 65-74 age group was consistent in all the practices surveyed and seems to be accounted for by the less frequent occurrence of stress incontinence in the older age groups. This was previously also noted by Brocklehurst et al.[7] The prevalence of urge incontinence alone was similar between the ages of 15 and 54 but increased after this age.

Figure 14.2 shows the results by parity in those aged 15 or over according to the type of urinary incontinence. Even in this large survey, the numbers with sub-categories of urinary incontinence in different parity groups are sometimes small, and some caution is therefore necessary in interpreting the results. Urinary incontinence was reported less commonly by nulliparous than parous women at all ages but, except in the age group 45-54, was no more common in those who had

Table 14.6: Community Prevalence of Urinary Incontinence in Boys

Age (years)	Never incontinent (%)	Occasionally incontinent (%)	Regularly incontinent (%)	Uncertain (%) replies	Total (100%)
5	64 (60)	24 (22)	19 (18)	0 (0)	107
6	112 (67)	33 (20)	18 (11)	4 (2)	167
7	124 (74)	25 (15)	15 (9)	3 (2)	167
8	115 (78)	18 (12)	12 (8)	2 (1)	147
9	136 (79)	19 (11)	15 (9)	2 (1)	172
10	142 (80)	21 (12)	12 (7)	2 (1)	177
11	148 (79)	23 (12)	15 (8)	1 (1)	187
12	177 (96)	5 (3)	2 (1)	1 (1)	185
13	158 (92)	7 (4)	5 (3)	2 (1)	172
14	189 (94)	9 (5)	3 (1)	0 (0)	201
Not known	2 (100)	0 (0)	0 (0)	0 (0)	0
Total	1367 (81)	185 (11)	116 (7)	17 (1)	1684

Table 14.7: Community Prevalence of Urinary Incontinence in Girls

Age (years)	Never incontinent (%)	Occasionally incontinent (%)	Regularly incontinent (%)	Uncertain (%) replies	Total (100%)
5	87 (68)	23 (18)	16 (12)	2 (2)	128
6	102 (71)	32 (22)	10 (7)	0 (0)	144
7	98 (72)	24 (18)	11 (8)	3 (2)	136
8	118 (80)	21 (14)	8 (5)	1 (1)	148
9	132 (85)	15 (10)	7 (4)	2 (1)	156
10	125 (82)	16 (10)	8 (5)	4 (1)	153
11	146 (89)	12 (7)	4 (2)	3 (2)	165
12	143 (89)	10 (6)	6 (4)	1 (1)	160
13	164 (92)	8 (4)	5 (3)	1 (1)	178
14	166 (90)	14 (8)	5 (3)	0 (0)	185
Not known	3 (100)	0 (0)	0 (0)	0 (0)	3
Total	1284 (83)	175 (11)	80 (5)	17 (1)	1556

Figure 14.1: The Prevalence of Stress, Urge and Stress/Urge Incontinence in Women by Age

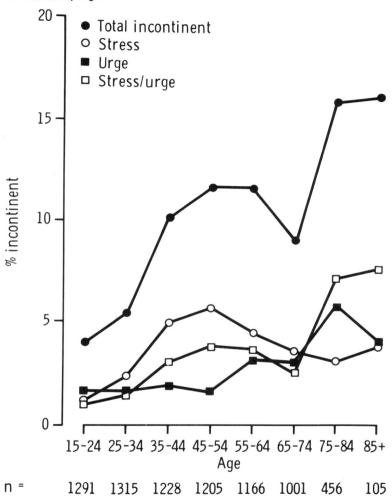

had four or more babies were most likely to report regular urinary incontinence. Urge incontinence may be a little commoner in the parous than the nulliparous, but within the parous there is no obvious increase in the prevalence of urge incontinence with increasing parity. The rise in the prevalence of incontinence with parity is due to a rise in the prevalence of stress (and stress/urge incontinence). The effects of parity on the prevalence of urinary incontinence are independent of the effects of age.

Figure 14.2: The Prevalence of Stress, Urge and Stress/Urge Incontinence in Women by Parity

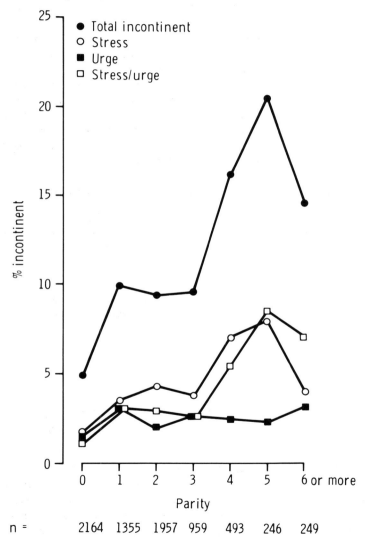

Information about patients' social class and ethnic origin was available in two of the practices surveyed and it was, therefore, possible to analyse the results to see if there were any differences between the prevalence of incontinence according to social class or ethnic group. (For these analyses a scoring system was used for urinary incontinence to include all categories of response — never = 0, uncertain = ½, occasional = 1, regular = 2. Mean incontinence rates for each group were calculated and compared.) After allowance for age differences, no significant differences were found between social classes for either sex. There were, however, some differences between the ethnic groups, after allowance for age. These are shown in Figure 14.3. Two main factors contributed to the ethnic group differences. These were a relative deficiency of urinary incontinence among women of Asian background (viz. those who were of Asian or part Asian parentage or grandparentage) and a relative excess of urinary incontinence amongst men of Afro Caribbean or part Afro Caribbean background.

Figure 14.3: Incontinence Rates According to Ethnic Background

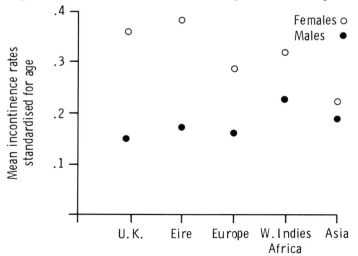

In two of the practices surveyed, those who had replied that they were regularly incontinent of urine were asked to agree to an interview by a nurse from the survey team. The same structured questionnaire as was used for those with recognised incontinence was administered. In addition the severity of incontinence was assessed using four possible categories:

Minimal: No extra laundry; no pads or expenses; no restrictions in activities because of incontinence.

Slight: Very small amount of extra laundry; pads worn only occasionally; no restriction in activities.

Moderate: Extra laundry or pads or expenses; some restriction in activities.

Severe: Extra laundry or pads or expenses; activities restricted; required help from others.

One hundred and seventy-eight (75 per cent) of the 237 adults approached were interviewed of whom twenty (11 per cent) were not confirmed to be incontinent of urine at interview. Of these, ten had had a temporary cause for their urinary incontinence at the time of the postal survey, three were incontinent only occasionally and seven had apparently made a mistake in completing the form.

One hundred and forty-nine (94 per cent) of those incontinent at interview said they had been incontinent for more than a year.

Table 14.8 shows the severity of urinary incontinence at first interview compared with that at follow-up in the 138 people who were interviewed twice. Few of those with minimal or slight incontinence at first interview considered themselves to have a problem warranting medical attention. Indeed almost all were incapacitated very little by the symptom. This seems to be a group for whom measures such as advice on obesity, pelvic floor exercises or explanation of bladder function may be relevant but offers of active medical investigation and management are not. Of those with moderate or severe incontinence, however, most were considerably handicapped by their symptoms and found them extremely embarrassing. Only two of the nine elderly in this group were not receiving help with incontinence management from local community services compared with 22 of the 25 aged under 65. Although not all of those not receiving these services would necessarily have welcomed or benefited from them, there did seem to be a gap between the number of incontinent people warranting services and those receiving them.

However, even when services were being provided there was still considerable room for improved continence management in many of those referred.

Of the 20 women with moderate or severe urinary incontinence initially, 15 patients (75 per cent) were in the same category after a year. The only changes at follow-up were improvements in five women, all in the 15-64 age group, two of whom had improved with

Table 14.8: Severity of Urinary Incontinence at First Interview Compared with Severity at One Year Follow-up

	First Interview				
	Severe	Moderate	Slight	Minimal	Total
Severe	12	0	• 0	2	14
Moderate	0	12	2	4	18
Slight	0	0	24	5	29
Minimal	0	3	5	43	51
Not incontinent	0	2	10	14	26
Total	12	17	41	68	138

no treatment. Of the 90 patients with minimal or slight incontinence initially, 57 (63 per cent) were in exactly the same category a year later. In 10 patients (11 per cent) the incontinence was more severe. Four (4 per cent) had improved and 19 (21 per cent) were no longer incontinent. Seven (37 per cent) of those no longer incontinent had had no treatment. Fewer of those aged 65 and over (1/25) had improved than that of the younger women (6/85) and only one of the 65 and over age group was no longer incontinent. Overall, therefore, there was no evidence that the symptom progressed or worsened in the space of a year in the majority of patients.

Faecal and Double Incontinence

Table 14.9 shows the results of the postal survey together with the number of patients interviewed and the number of those whose faecal incontinence was confirmed at interview. Interviews were carried out with 66 (65 per cent) of the 101 adults reporting faecal or double incontinence in two of the practices. When the letter requesting an interview was sent out some requests were refused on the grounds that the positive reply had referred only to very minor staining associated with constipation or haemorrhoids. This, and the very personal nature of the symptom, probably accounts for the response rate of only 65 per cent. As a result of these replies to the request for interview and from the interviews it was clear that the unconfirmed postal survey results were likely to be an overestimate of the prevalence of faecal and double incontinence. The prevalence of faecal incontinence is thus based on the proportion of patients in each age/sex group whose faecal incontinence was confirmed at interview. It was not felt justifiable to approach a sample of those who had reported no faecal incontinence to try to validate these negative answers.

Table 14.9: Community Prevalence of Faecal or Double Incontinence

Age/Sex	Faecal incontinence reported at postal survey	Numbers interviewed (two practices)	Faecal incontinence confirmed	Estimated prevalence of faecal and double incontinence (per 1,000)
15-64 Male (n=5975)	58	14	6	4.2
65 + (n=1102)	45	15	4	10.9
15-64 Female (n=6205)	63	24	4	1.7
65 + (n=1562)	45	13	6	13.3
Total (n=14844)	211	66	20	4.3

Of the 20 people whose faecal incontinence was confirmed at interview only three were receiving help from community nurses or social workers, or from pad or laundry services. Eleven had not told their general practitioner of the problem. Two of the six men aged 15-64 and two of the four men aged 65 and over were doubly incontinent as was one of the four women aged 15-64 and all six of the women aged 65 and over. Thus, nine patients were identified with isolated faecal incontinence. Six of these had relatively minor problems, usually staining associated with constipation or haemorrhoids, while three men (aged 39, 52 and 70) had severe continuing faecal incontinence.

Conclusions

These surveys have confirmed previous findings that incontinence is a common symptom for which medical or other help may not be sought. Although minor degrees of even regular incontinence are often not regarded as a problem, in its more severe form the symptom causes a considerable degree of handicap to the sufferer and often to carers as well. There is no doubt that there is a substantial group of incontinent people of all ages who would benefit from investigation and active treatment as well as those for whom management measures such as appliances, pads and pants or home adaptations would improve their quality of life.

In addition, however, the services currently being used by incontinent people need to be kept constantly under review. Services being provided for the incontinent may not be being deployed in the most efficient and beneficial way.

Improved education of professionals and public, a health district based incontinence service and rigorous evaluation of equipment, treatment and services would help ensure that all incontinent people receive optimum management.[19]

Notes

1. Rutter, M., Yule, W. and Graham, P. (1973), 'Enuresis and Behavioural Deviance: Some Epidemiological Considerations' in Kolvin, I., MacKeith, R.C. (eds) *Bladder Control and Enuresis* (Heinemann, London), 137-47 (Clinics in Developmental Medicine nos. 48/9).
2. Wolin, L.H. (1969), 'Stress Incontinence in Young Healthy Nulliparous Female Subjects', *Brit. J. Urol.*, *101*, 545-9.

3. Nemir, A. and Middleton, R.P. (1954), 'Stress Incontinence in Young Nulliparous Women', *Amer. J. Gynec.*, *68*, 1166-8.

4. Crist, T., Shingleton, H.M. and Kock, G.G. (1971), 'Stress Incontinence in the Nulliparous Patients', *Obst. Gynec.*, *40*, 13-7.

5. Osborne, J.L. (1976), 'Post-menopausal Changes in Micturition Habits and in Urine Flow and Urethral Pressure Studies' in Campbell, S. (ed.) *The Management of the Menopause and Post-menopausal Years*, MTP, Lancaster, 285-9.

6. Brocklehurst, J.C., Fry, J., Griffiths, L.L. and Kalton, G. (1972), 'Urinary Infection and Symptoms of Dysuria in Women Aged 45-65 Years: Their Relevance to Similar Findings in the Elderly', *Age Ageing*, *1*, 41-7.

7. Knox, J.D.E. (1979), 'Ambulant Incontinent Patients in General Practice. A survey to ascertain the prevalence of these patients and their distribution by type of practice', *Nursing Times*, *75*, 1683.

8. Brocklehurst, J.C., Dillane, J.B., Griffiths, L. and Fry, J. (1968), 'The Prevalence and Symptomatology of Urinary Infection in an Aged Population', *Gerontology*, *10*, 242-53.

9. Milne, J.S., Williamson, J., Maule, M.M. and Wallace, E.T. (1972), 'Urinary Symptoms in Older People', *Modern Geriatrics*, *2*, 198-212.

10. Yarnell, J.W.G. and St Leger, A.S. (1979), 'The Prevalence, Severity and Factors Associated with Urinary Incontinence in a Random Sample of the Elderly', *Age Ageing*, *8*, 81-5.

11. Isaacs, B. and Walkey, F.A. (1964), 'A Survey of Incontinence in Elderly Hospital Patients', *Gerontology*, *6*, 367-76.

12. McLaren, S.M., McPherson, F.M., Sinclair, F. and Ballinger, B.R. (1981), 'Prevalence and Severity of Incontinence among Hospitalised, Female Psychogeriatric Patients', *Health Bull.*, *39*, 157.

13. Brocklehurst, J.C. (1972), 'Bowel Management in the Neurologically Disabled. The problems of old age', *Proc. R. Soc. Med.*, *65*, 66; *Sec. Proctology*, 2-5.

14. Thomas, T.M., Plymat, K.R., Blannin, J. and Meade, T.W. (1980), 'Prevalence of Urinary Incontinence', *Brit. Med. J.*, *281*, 1243-5.

15. Thomas, T.M., Egan, M., Walgrove, A. and Meade, T.W. (1984), 'The Prevalence of Faecal and Double Incontinence', *Community Medicine*, *6*, 216-20.

16. Thomas, T.M., Karran, O.D. and Meade, T.W. (1981), 'Management of Urinary Incontinence in Patients with Multiple Sclerosis', *J. Roy. Coll. of Gen. Practs.*, *31*, 296-8.

17. Townsend, J., Heng, L., Thomas, T.M., Egan, M. and Meade, T.W. (1981), 'Costs of Incontinence to Families with Severely Handicapped Children', *Community Medicine*, *3*, 119-22.

18. Egan, M., Plymat, K., Thomas, T.M. and Meade, T.W. (1983), 'Incontinence in Patients in Two General Hospitals, *Nursing Mirror*, 2 Feb.

19. Kings Fund project paper (1983), 'Action on Incontinence. Report of a working group', no. 43.

APPENDIX A: GUIDELINES ON THE ROLE OF THE DISTRICT CONTINENCE ADVISER

Compiled by the Executive Committee, The Association of Continence Advisers, March 1985

The Continence Adviser

1. Introduction

Only recently has continence advising attained widespread recognition as a nursing speciality in its own right. Its pioneers came from a wide range of disciplines and few held posts specifically concerned with caring for incontinent people. Little or no formal education on the subject was available to them and expertise grew, largely by trial and error, from a determination to do something more positive for this large group of people.

Today, this situation is changing rapidly and many health districts are appointing continence advisers to specially created posts. However, no formal guidelines exist, at present, to help appointers and new appointees to plan, establish and run a continence advisory service. It is primarily for them that this document has been produced. It is also hoped that it will be of help to those already running a service but wanting to develop it.

2. The Post

The primary function of the continence adviser is to promote continence by providing an educational/advisory service for professionals and others caring for the incontinent person.

The post will require a senior nurse (such as Sister I), accountable to the District Nursing Officer or Chief Nursing Officer. He or she will be expected to take, or to have taken English National Board Course No. 978: 'An Introduction to Promotion of Continence and Management of Incontinence'. Membership of the Association of Continence Advisers would also be of great value.

3. Job Description

The broad objective of the new appointee will be to plan the service. It will be necessary to identify current needs and resources in the district. This will be best achieved by making personal contact with those in the district concerned with incontinence in a nursing, medical, paramedical and administrative capacity. Different people will be involved in each district but the following is offered as a suggested checklist:

1. Nursing:
   — Directors of nursing services
   — Directors of nurse education
   — District nurse tutors (college-based)
   — Community and ward nursing staff.
2. Medical:
   — Consultants (and their staff) in the relevant medical specialities, e.g. geriatric medicine, urology, gynaecology and paediatrics
   — Local general practitioners' committee.
3. Paramedical:
   — District physiotherapist and staff
   — District occupational therapist and staff
   — Director of social services (hospital social worker) and staff
   — Local and hospital pharmacists
   — Firms offering an aids fitting service.
4. Administration:
   — Administrators
   — Supplies officers
   — Finance officers.

Contact should also be made with other local continence advisers, or specially designated nurses, and the local health education unit if one exists.

The role of the continence adviser is a very isolated one and it is useful to form a supportive working party — consisting of people from the above list — to help with the setting up of the service and its ongoing evaluation.

The responsibilities of the adviser will include clinical, educational and administrative roles as well as acting as a co-ordinator of services. The detailed nature of the job will depend on local circumstances and it may take many months for the new appointee to become effective in all aspects of his or her role.

3.1 Clinical. In conjunction with medical personnel, it will be necessary to provide a regular specialist service/clinic for the assessment of incontinent patients where suitable forms of treatment and management can be agreed. It is not advisable for the continence adviser to carry a personal case load but rather to provide specialist input to those immediately caring for patients. Experience has shown that it otherwise becomes impossible to function adequately in other important aspects of the job.

It may be appropriate to be involved in joint domiciliary visits with members of the primary health care team. In some districts there will be involvement with a urodynamic service but this should only be in a supporting role to the consultant in charge.

3.2 Self Education. An introductory period of self-education is essential but to remain an effective educator the adviser must continue to keep abreast of advances in this rapidly developing field. Self-education will happen informally through reading and practical experience but it will also be invaluable to attend courses and conferences whenever possible and to visit advisers in other districts.

3.3 Educational. The primary aim of the continence adviser will be to promote continence by education of nursing colleagues (pre- and post-registration), and other professionals concerned with patient care. Teaching may need to be extended to supporting relatives, and community-based groups.

Most of the adviser's role as an educator will involve him or her being available for informal advice by phone, letter, or in person. Knowledge and information can be disseminated through study days, seminars and informal teaching. The adviser may be asked to teach on ENB and statutory district nurse courses as well as running training schemes for social workers, home helps and others.

To be an effective adviser it will be necessary to establish and maintain a body of information so that enquiries can be dealt with efficiently. Suggested ways of doing this would be: (a) keeping abreast of nursing and other specialist journals, books and leaflets; (b) keeping up to date with new therapies and incontinence management techniques; and (c) gathering and indexing information as it becomes available (e.g. from the DHSS, the Incontinence Advisory Service at the Disabled Living Foundation, the Association of Continence Advisers and manufacturers of aids) and disseminating it to those who could benefit.

3.4 Liaison/Co-ordination. The continence adviser will be the natural focus for promoting continence in the district and as such will have a valuable role as a co-ordinator of effort and a liaison person.

It will be necessary to establish working links with such people as: supplies and finance officers, administrators, purchasing advisory groups, linen service managers and environmental health officers.

Regular meetings with link or resource nurses from such areas as obstetrics, surgery, medicine, paediatrics, mental handicap and mental illness from hospital and community will provide a forum for ready discussion and dissemination of information.

It will also be fruitful to maintain contact with manufacturers of aids to discuss consumer needs and future developments.

3.5 Administration. Accurate documentation must be kept. This will include nursing records, teaching commitments, manufacturers' visits, and aids and equipment available within the district.

There will also be administrative work to be done in maintaining an information service, and arranging meetings and the like.

3.6 Evaluation/Research. When new therapies and management techniques and equipment become available the adviser will be well placed to initiate and co-ordinate trials and evaluations. Information from such work should be relayed to the supplies system and any other interested parties in the district.

4. Practical Requirements

When appointing an adviser it will be necessary to know what his or her practical requirements will be. A realistic budget would take account of: office space; a direct telephone/answerphone; teaching expenses; educational material and, above all, clerical assistance.

APPENDIX B: CHECKLISTS AND GUIDELINES FOR PROFESSIONAL STAFF

Dorothy Mandelstam

(1) Urinary Incontinence

There are a number of different manifestations of abnormal bladder function, some of which result in incontinence. When this occurs, understanding of the type and form influences management. Answers to the following questions, put to the patient sympathetically and in private, will be a useful guide:

(1) How long have you been troubled in this way?
(2) Did it start suddenly or gradually? Was it associated with any particular event?
(3) Do you feel the need to pass urine more frequently than usual during the day? How often? And also at night? How often? Are you drinking more fluid than usual?
(4) Do you have a feeling of urgency? How much warning time do you get? Do you ever have an 'accident'? (Urge incontinence.)
(5) Do you wet yourself without being aware of passing urine? Is the leakage a little or a lot? (Retention with overflow incontinence; reflex emptying.)
(6) Do you have a small leakage of urine on slight exertion, such as coughing or sneezing or laughing, or even turning over in bed? (Stress incontinence.) Or is the leakage on exertion considerable? (Unstable bladder and stress incontinence.)
(7) Do you dribble just after having passed urine?

If necessary, the information obtained can be verified and expanded by talking separately, and out of hearing of the patient, to relatives and other members of staff.

The Promotion of Continence

Observation and charting of the pattern of micturition of the patient is necessary, over a week or longer, as well as a note of the pattern of micturition before admission. The patient at home can be asked to fill in a simple chart.

Where the patient is incontinent but aware of the need to micturate, attention to environmental factors can help to re-establish and maintain continence. The following need to be looked at:

(1) What does the pattern of micturition show, and is the existing toilet routine frequent enough for the patient's needs? Can the patient indicate these needs? (If aphasic this is especially important.) Stroke patients may also require visual retraining in relation to toilet facilities.

(2) Are adequate toilet facilities, whether lavatory, commode or urinal, available and readily accessible? Relative heights of bed, chair and commode are important, as well as the type and positioning of the commode. Warmth and privacy are essential. Can clothing be managed quickly and easily?

(3) If the patient is on diuretics, are they being administered at the most suitable time? Are they still necessary?

(4) Is there a reasonable fluid intake during the day? Is there need to restrict drinks two or three hours before sleep?

(5) Is nightime sedation impairing awareness of the need to micturate and so causing bed-wetting?

(6) Is the patient constipated? Constipation leading to faecal impaction is a common cause of both urinary and faecal incontinence (spurious diarrhoea) in the elderly.

On the basis of information so far gathered, consideration can now also be given to the possibility of habit retraining, where appropriate. This differs from rigid toiletting (see[1,2]).

Management of Incontinence

Where certain forms of incontinence are not amenable to treatment (apart from routine rigid toiletting) personal protection is essential. The type of protection used will depend on:

(1) the amount and occasion of leakage, whether during the day or night, and whether when up and dressed, or in bed; and

(2) the age and physical and mental condition of the patient, and the degree of mobility and dexterity.

Pads and Pants. There is a wide variety available, and choice depends on individual needs. They are:

(1) based on different principles;
(2) of differing degrees of absorbency; and
(3) of different designs.

They are used mainly by women, but may be appropriate for some men. Supply should be through Area Health Authorities supplies departments, although range may be limited. Private supply (mainly by mail order) is an alternative.

Urinary Appliances. These are available for men, but most types need to be chosen and fitted individually. Some hospitals provide a skilled fitting service, and certain large firms of medical suppliers can also fit and supply on prescription.

Long-term Catheterisation (for intractable incontinence). The use of a catheter (a joint medical/nursing/patient decision) may permit more independence, for instance to live at home. Drainage into a leg-bag, or a bag supported and concealed in a waist-belt, enables the patient to lead a fairly active daily life.

Underpads. If these are used, are they of sufficient size and absorbency? Are they positioned correctly, i.e. across the bed and not lengthwise?

Laundry and Supply/Disposal Services. For the patient at home, are these services provided, and are they adequate?

Notes

1. Clay, E.C. (1978), 'Incontinence of Urine', *Nursing Mirror* (2, 9, 16 and 23 March).
2. Browne, B. (1978), *Management for Continence* (Age Concern, London).

Management of Bowels

Bowel activity or actions can be a source of worry to patients. In order to alleviate these worries and prevent distress and constipation, or worse still faecal incontinence, time spent with the patient on admission to find out normal habits is of value. The following points need to be considered:

(1) How regular is the normal bowel habit? This can vary from three times a day to three times a week. A record is necessary of

frequency, nature and number of stools and if there is pain or discomfort on defaecation.

(2) When were the bowels last opened?

(3) Is the bowel stimulated by any particular event, such as a glass of hot water first or last thing?

(4) Is there a history of use of laxatives? Are any constipating drugs being taken, such as analgesics, hypnotics, iron, etc?

(5) Should diet be considered? A new environment and sedentary existence, unaccustomed diet, limitation of fluid intake and so on may affect bowel habits.

(6) Are toilet facilities adequate in numbers, appropriate in type and readily accessible? Are there sufficient number of commodes for night and emergency use and are they of the right design?

(7) If feasible can lavatory or commode be used instead of bedpan? The latter is difficult to use and can lead to excess straining.

(8) Whatever toilet facility is used, is it available at the time of need and can it be used with privacy? Lack of privacy is inhibiting and distressing. Are there locks on the lavatory doors?

(9) How does the patient communicate need to defaecate, particularly if aphasic, unable to speak much English or extremely shy?

(10) Can patient wash hands or can wipes be provided?

(11) If faecal incontinence exists is it due to faecal impaction? This is very common in elderly people. After disimpaction minimal dosage of aperients should be used to restore regular emptying of the rectum. Type and dosage need to be given to the type of food acceptable to the patient and of sufficient fibre content, and the giving of adequate fluids.

(12) Continued observation is required to note any change in bowel habit.

The following is a list of different types of therapeutic agents and their function.

(1) Hydrophilic bulking agents — dietary fibre (wholemeal bread)
　　　　　　　　　　　　　　　　　bran fibre
　　　　　　　　　　　　　　　　　pharmaceutical preparations, e.g.
　　　　　　　　　　　　　　　　　Fybogel, Isogel, Normacol
Function — to supplement a diet that is inadequate in satisfying the volume requirements of the gut.

(2) Chemical laxatives — Bisacodyl — Dulcolax
　　　　　　　　　　　　Senna aglycone — Senokot
Function — to act on the colon to stimulate peristalsis.

(3) Rectal evacuants — large or small normal saline
   (a) washouts
   (b) retention enemas — vegetable oil
                              dioctyl sodium
                              sulphosuccinate
   (c) disposable enemas — Fletchers
                              Fleet
      foaming enema   — (if available)
   (d) suppositories, e.g. Dulocolax
                              glycerine
                              Beogex
      foaming suppositories
Function — to evacuate impacted faeces or to affect clearance of bowel prior to surgery, radiology, etc. in situations where oral laxatives are not effective.

Faecal Incontinence

Faecal incontinence, although it occurs less frequently than urinary incontinence, is more distressing to patients and relatives, and often not so easily tolerated by nursing staff. The action of the bowel, however, can often be more successfully controlled than that of the bladder. Despite many people's life-long preoccupation with their bowels, they usually have little understanding of the physiology of digestion and excretion, and so harmful habits persist like prolonged straining (sometimes from childhood) which can give rise to problems later in life. On admission to hospital the situation is often made worse by routine procedures and practices followed without regard to the individual patient's own bowel habits.

Normal Physiology

The requirements of a normal bowel action are an alimentary tract with nerve and blood supply, and stimuli which promote the functioning and co-ordination of smooth and striated muscle, to produce a downward movement of the bowel contents.

The Colon

The residual waste products of digestion accumulate in the colon, where absorption of water occurs. Colonic movement (smooth muscle activity) consists of segmentation and peristalsis. The movement of the contents of the colon by peristaltic activity occurs many times during the day stimulated by reflexes such as the gastro-colic reflexes.

Transit

The rate at which the content passes through the alimentary tract is variable; most time is taken up with passage through the colon. The total time has been shown to be on average 96 hours but there is wide variation between individuals (sometimes as short as 6–12 hours).

The Rectum

The rectum, the reservoir for faeces, is normally involved in continence and defaecation. There is a valve-like mechanism at the ano-rectal junction which helps prevent the flow of faeces into the anal canal until an appropriate time. The competence of this mechanism depends on the tone of the pubo-rectalis muscle producing the angle which the rectum forms with the anal canal. This angle is maintained by pubo-rectalis, a muscle of the pelvic floor. The pelvic muscles react reflexively in response to changes in intra-abdominal pressure in addition to any change of pressure or volume within the rectum. It is probable that rectal sensation is registered by receptors in the levatores ani-muscles and not in the rectal wall itself (Parks, 1975) as the rectum is closely related to the pelvic floor for much of its length. It can be seen that laxity of the pelvic floor muscles may have implications in relation to ano-rectal continence. While their reflex actions are automatic, they can also be contracted voluntarily and their efficiency increased (see previous section), and this is important in some cases.

Anal Canal

There is a ring of voluntary muslces surrounding the end of the alimentary tract, the circular muscle of the bowel wall having become thickened to form the internal sphincter. The lining of the anal canal is very sensitive to touch and pressure. These muscles and the sensitive anal canal lining play some part in faecal continence. The surrounding muscles can be strengthened if necessary by active exercise in conjunction with the pelvic floor, providing that the nerve supply to it is normal.

Factors Affecting Mobility in the Colon

A number of factors influence colonic movement and therefore have a direct bearing on bowel management:

(1) Changes in posture from lying, sitting or standing affect pressure in the alimentary tract. Pressure waves in the colon may result from alteration of tone in the abdominal muscles, as well as from physical movement.

(2) Food: the gastro-colic reflexes are initiated by eating, resulting in increased motor activity in the alimentary tract. The ileum discharges its contents into the colon stimulating activity along the whole colon. These responses can also be induced by the sight or smell of food.

(3) Emotions: it is well known that bowel habits can be affected by emotional stress although the actual mechanism by which the colon is affected is unknown. Conditioning in childhood, and social factors, can sometimes produce eccentric patterns of behaviour in relation to bowel action, and so does anxiety about 'normal' bowel functions.

Normal Bowel Habit

Normal habit is specific to the individual and there is great variation. Although the majority of people appear to have a motion every day, it is now recognised that bowel frequency can range from three actions a week to three actions a day (Connell *et al.*, 1965). The picture of normal defaecation in a subject depends on information not only about frequency but volume and consistency of stool. For instance, a very small stool passed daily with great strain is not normal, and neither is persistent urgency, even though the frequency pattern might be normal. All these factors require detailed attention on admission to hospital, where change of routine and diet can upset the patient and lead to constipation and even faecal impaction which may present as incontinence. Mechanical and psychological difficulties arising from the use of bedpans, commodes, lack of privacy, are contributory factors.

Causes of Faecal Incontinence

(1) Faecal impaction — this is one of the most common causes, particularly in elderly and immobile people. Impaction can result from neglect of call to stool, diminished awareness of the feeling of a full rectal feeble peristaltic movement, incomplete evacuation and impairment of the mechanism of defaecation. Faeces accumulating in the rectum or colon can become dehydrated and compacted, leading to the passage of more fluid stools seeping past the impacted mass (spurious diarrhoea seepage).

(2) Persistent diarrhoea has many causes and medical opinion is essential. Some causes such as excessive use of purgatives, bowel infections, or functional disorder producing a colitis, may lead to incontinence.

(3) Trauma — incontinence may follow anatomical distortion from childbirth or surgery or injury. It may also accompany rectal prolapse. In some women incontinence is due to a defective ano-rectal muscle ring producing faulty valve function. Spinal injury with loss of ano-rectal sensation and impaired muscle function can lead to faecal incontinence, though many of these cases can be controlled.

(4) Patients with brain lesions or dementia may be unaware of the urge of sensation of defaecation; if so a formed stool is passed without their knowledge.

Treatment of Faecal Incontinence

Faecal Impaction

It must be emphasised that this condition is preventable, and it should never be allowed to arise on admission to hospital. The following preventive routine is suggested:

(1) The nurse needs to spend time with the patient or relative to ascertain the bowel pattern before admission, and any special methods of maintaining it, e.g. diet, glass of warm water, smoking, etc.

(2) Recording of bowel actions and conservation of stool are needed, noting the frequency, consistency and bulk.

(3) Consideration should be given to the effects of any drugs prescribed, e.g. analgesics, sedatives, tranquillisers, etc.

(4) Frequently in hospital, laxatives are necessary to prevent constipation, e.g. Senokot, which stimulates the smooth muscles of the colon, Milpar, or Dobanex; without any obvious adverse effects. Over a period of one or two weeks the dose can be adjusted to determine the smallest effective amount. It is even more important to ensure that the diet contains adequate roughage, that there is a good fluid intake and as much physical activity as possible.

(5) Adequate lavatory facilities, or their substitutes, are necessary. Defaecation is easier in the sitting position; a bedpan should only be used if absolutely necessary; it is now known that it involves a greater degree of straining than normal defaecation.

This has significance for patients with cardio-vascular disease (Halpern, 1960). Whatever receptacle is used, privacy and warmth must be ensured. There should be toilet paper within easy reach of the user, particularly for hemiplegic patients. Patients naturally prefer to use the lavatory, even if they have to be wheeled there. They also like to be able to lock the door. Many hospitals have too few lavatories, in spite of official recommendations as far back as 1961 that there should be one per six patients, with enough space to accommodate wheelchairs (Ministry of Health Building Notes).

Treatment of Faecal Impaction

Faecal impaction, although readily identified, is often overlooked as the rectal examination unfortunately is all too often omitted. The main aim of treatment is to evacuate the faecal contents and prevent recurring impaction. There are two types of impaction:

(1) Scybalous: consisting of hard faeces in the rectum.
(2) Pultaceous: putty-like faeces in the distal colon.

Treatment of Scybalous Types. A number of motions are necessary in order to clear the bowel, and enemas and suppositories may be required on successive days. Clearance needs to be confirmed by repeated digital examinations. If removal of faeces needs to be immediate, digital evacuation is effective. This can usually be carried out on the ward, and very rarely requires a general anaesthetic. The use of a local anaesthetic and lubricating gel makes this process less uncomfortable for the patient.

Treatment of Pultaceous Type. This is less common and oral laxatives can be used, with suppositories and enemas. The use of Senokot, particularly in granule form has been found successful. In both types after the bowel is emptied and during the restorative period oral laxatives or suppositories may be required to initiate defaecation. To avoid future impaction, the particular circumstances which led to its existence must not be allowed to recur. Attention must be paid to diet to ensure adequate fibre content. An increase in fluid intake is required. The use of bulk formers such as Isogel, Normacol or bran are recommended.

Severe Diarrhoea

Medical investigation is essential. In some cases of persistent and intractable incontinence, pads and pants may be needed.

Surgery

This is indicated in a number of cases of ano-rectal incontinence. When obstetrical injury to the external anal sphincter occurs, the sphincter may be repaired directly, by overlapping the two ends of the torn muscle. However, when incontinence occurs as a result of congenital defects, rectal prolapse or following nerve damage (Parks, Swash, Urlich, 1977), a post-anal repair may be necessary. This involves the lacing up of the pelvic floor behind the rectum and restoration of the ano-rectal angle (Parks, Presidential Address, Royal Society of Medicine, 1975). Nerve damage may result from trauma following stretching of the pudendal nerves during a long labour, the use of high forceps, or during prolonged straining at defaecation over many years (Parks, Swash, Urlich, 1977).

Spinal Injury

Incontinence can be avoided by planned evacuation at suitable times. This involves inducing a state of mild constipation by suitable diet and instigating bowel activity by the use of suppositories or enemas or manual stimulation.

Brain Damage

Incontinence due to brain damage can be controlled by the planned use of laxatives at night, aimed to empty the bowel in the morning, while drugs known to have constipating effects are used during the day. Regular washouts two or three times a week may be needed.

Laxatives, Suppositories and Enemas

These should be prescribed by the doctor, following consultation with nursing staff, and dosage and effects should then be monitored jointly. Laxatives are useful in softening the stool and stimulating colon activity, and suppositories stimulate rectal and colonic activity and precipitate defaecation. Enemas add fluid to the colonic contents, and stimulate colonic activity. Soap enemas are now thought to be undesirable. However, there are now many types of enemas available, as well as warm oil enemas, that are also effective. Colonic washouts are also valuable. Care should be taken to prevent damage to the mucosa of the rectum and even perforation of the bowel when administering an enema. When the enema has been administered it needs to be retained by the patient for 10 minutes or so to be effective.

References

Parks, A.G. (Nov. 1975), Proceedings Royal Society of Medicine, vol. 68, no. 11, 681-90.

Connell, A.M., Hilton, C., Lennard-Jones, J.E. and Misciewicz, J.J. (1965), 'Variation of Bowel Habit in Two Population Samples', *Brit. Med. J.*, *2*, 1095-9.

Halpern, A., Shaftel, N., Selman, D., Shaftel, H., Kuhn, P.H., Samuels, S.S. and Birch, H.G. (1960), 'The Straining Forces of a Bowel Function', *Angiology*, 426-42.

Parks, A.G., Swash, M. and Urlich, H. (1977), 'Sphincter Denervation in Anorectal Incontinence and Rectal Prolapse', *Gut*, *18*, 656-65.

Further Reading

Wright, L. (1974), 'Bowel Function in Hospital Patients', Nursing Care Project Reports, Series 1, no. 4 (RCN, London).

Avery Jones, Sir Francis and Godding, E. (eds) (1972), *Management of Constipation* (Blackwell).

These notes on faecal incontinence have been prepared by Dorothy Mandelstam, with acknowledgements to Mr Michael Niell, FRACS, lately Research Fellow, St Mark's Hospital, London.

APPENDIX C: EQUIPMENT

In the United Kingdom incontinence aids (with one or two exceptions) are not on prescription. Supply can often be arranged through other channels in the National Health Service, but choice is limited by shortage of information about what is available and appropriate. For this reason a list of the items of equipment mentioned in the text of this book (particularly Chapter 9) follows. Names and addresses of manufacturers are given, from whom information can be requested. This list is not comprehensive, and many firms make similar products.

1. Kanga Pants and Pads (Figure C.1)	Nicholas Laboratories Ltd., 225 Bath Road, Slough, Berks SL1 4AU

Figure C.1

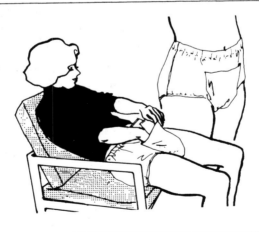

2. Tenaform Pants and Pads. (Figure C.2)	Molnlycke Ltd., Southfields Road, Dunstable, Beds LU6 3EJ

Figure C.2

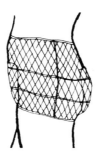

3. Pubic pressure urinal
   (many examples)

1. Charles S. Bullen Ltd.,
   3-7 Moss Street,
   Liverpool L6 1ET
2. Downs Surgical Ltd.,
   Church Path,
   Mitcham, Surrey CR4 3UE

4. Penile cone –
   McGuire Urinal 508

C.R. Bard International Ltd.,
Pennywell Industrial Estate,
Sunderland SR4 9EW

5. Sheath or condom urinals –
   Stoke Mandeville type.

1. Dept of Health & Social Security,
   Government Buildings,
   Warbreck Hill Road,
   Blackpool F72 0UZ
2. Downs Surgical Ltd.

6. Posey Sheath Holder

Martin Creasey Rehabilitation,
89, Clumber St.,
Hull HU5 3KH

7. Adhesive strip
   (double-sided)

Squibb Surgicare,
141-9 Staines Road,
Hounslow,
Middx TW3 3JB

Coloplast Ltd,
Bridge House,
Orchard Lane,
Huntingdon, Cambs PE18 6QT

8. Dow Corning Adhesive	Aldington Laboratories Ltd., Mersham, Ashford, Kent
9. Dribblet bag	Charles S. Bullen Ltd.
10. Pocket pad	Molnlycke Ltd.
11. Female catheter	C.R. Bard International Ltd.
12. Leg-bags	1. Seton Products Ltd., Tubiton House, Medlock Street. Oldham, OD1 3HS 2. C.R. Bard International Ltd.
13. Shepheard Sporran	Brevet Hospital Products, 16 Bridge Street, Caversham, Reading, Berks RG4 7AA
14. Inflatable occlusive device for men	Spencer Ltd, Spencer House, Britannia Road, Banbury, Oxon
15. Foam tampon	Rocket of London Ltd, Surgical Equipment, Imperial Way, Watford, Herts WD2 4XX
16. Edwards' Device	Raymed, a division of: Charles S. Thackray Ltd., 47 George Street, Leeds LS1 3BB
17. Bonnar's Device	Eschmann Bros & Walsh Ltd., Peter Road, Lancing, W. Sussex BN15 8TJ
18. Non-spill adaptor (Figure C.3)	Raymed (Charles S. Thackray Ltd.)

Figure C.3

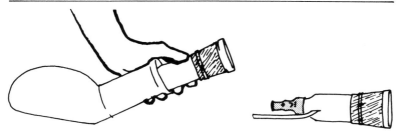

Figure C.4

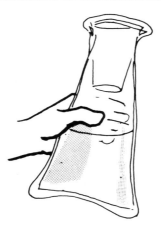

Figure C.5

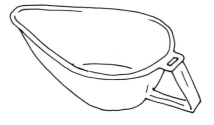

Figure C.6

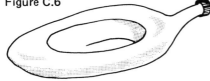

19. Reddy-bottle (Figure C.4)	Downs Surgical Ltd.
20. St Peter's Boat female urinal (Figure C.5)	Cape Warwick Ltd, Birmingham Road, Warwick CV34 4TX
21. Suba-Seal female urinal (code 5a 50) (Figure C.6)	William Freeman & Co Ltd., Suba-Seal Works, Staincross, Barnsley, Yorks S75 6DH
22. Feminal – personal female urinal. (Figure C.7)	Franklin Medical Ltd, Turnpike Road, Cressex Industrial Estate, High Wycombe, Bucks HP12 3NB

Figure C.7

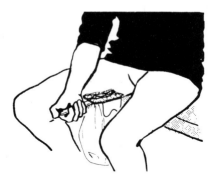

23. Kylie washable absorbent bed-sheet	Nicholas Laboratories Ltd., 225 Bath Road, Slough, Berks
24. Nilodor neutralising deodorant	Loxley Medical Supplies Ltd., Bessingby Industrial Estate, Bridlinton, North Humberside YO16 4SU

(Illustrations, by Brenda Naylor, are taken from Mandelstam, D. (1977), *Incontinence* (Heinemann Medical Books Ltd. on behalf of the Disabled Living Foundation, London), and are reproduced by kind permission.)

Commodes

There are many available — wooden-framed or tubular metal types, with and without arms. Seat heights vary and some tubular ones are adjustable. The commode should have a wide base for stability and, for the patient's ease of transfer, should be the same height as the chair or bed. Removable arms may be an advantage. If the patient's feet cannot rest flat on the floor (position aids defecation), a small foot-stool may be needed.

If the commode cannot be emptied immediately after use add Nilodor to prevent odour (see item 24 in this Appendix).

Other Toilet Problems

Whether a commode or lavatory is used, the following may need to be considered:

Can the person undress easily?

Consider clothing for quick removal and adjustment, special and adapted clothing.

Can he sit down and stand up safely?

Consider support rails beside lavatory and the possibility of raised lavatory seat (4"-6"). If in wheelchair consider method of transfer. If needed, place commode at right angles or less to front edge of chair. Patient who can stand can pivot round by rotating hips to sit on commode. If he cannot stand, removable commode arms will enable him to edge over on to commode.

Can he clean himself?	Adjust position of toilet paper to appropriate side if there is restricted use of arm or hand (stroke patient). Consider long-handled sponge, disposable wipes or bidet.
Can he wash his hands easily?	Consider washing facilities, e.g. hose on tap, bowl of water on chair or medicated wipes in foil or plastic container.

Further Information

The Incontinence Advisory Service, The Disabled Living Foundation, 380-384 Harrow Road, London W9 2HU provides through the incontinence adviser a specialised advisory and educational service on the subject of incontinence to professionals and the general public. It also produces up-to-date information on aids and equipment.

The Association of Continence Advisors (see Chapter 9), c/o the above address, has produced a Directory of Aids (incontinence) and a Directory of Aids to Toiletting.

FURTHER READING

Medical Textbooks

Brocklehurst, J.C. (ed.) (1978) *Textbook of Geriatric Medicine and Gerontology*, 2nd edn (Churchill Livingstone, Edinburgh)

Caldwell, K.P. (ed.) (1975) *Urinary Incontinence* (Sector Press, London)

Henry, M.M. and Swash, M. (eds.) (1985) *Coloproctology and the Pelvic Floor* (Butterworths, London and Boston)

Isaacs, B., Livingstone, M. and Neville, Y. (1972) *Survival of the Unfittest* (Routledge & Kegan Paul, London and Boston)

Stanton, S.L. (1977) *Female Urinary Incontinence* (Lloyd-Luke, London; Year Book, Chicago)

—— (ed.) (1984) *Clinical Gynecologic Urology* (C.V. Mosby Company, St Louis)

Willington, F.L. (ed.) (1976) *Incontinence in the Elderly* (Academic Press, London and New York)

Practical Handbooks

Browne, Bob (1978) *Management for Continence* (Age Concern, Mitcham, Surrey)

Burns, E.M., Isaacs, B. and Gracie, T. (1973) *Geriatric Nursing* (Heinemann, London)

Department of Health and Social Security (1979) *Aids for Disabled People. Evaluation of Personal Hygiene Needs* (HMSO, London)

Feneley, R.C.L. and Blannin, J.P. (1984) *Incontinence*, Patient Handbook Series, no. 18 (Churchill Livingstone, Edinburgh)

Hawker, M. (1974) *Geriatrics for Physiotherapists and the Allied Professions* (Faber and Faber, London)

—— (1978) *Return to Mobility* (Chest, Heart and Stroke Association, London)

Jay, P. (1974) *Coping with Disability* (Disabled Living Foundation, London)

Macartney, P. (1985) *Clothes Sense for Handicapped People of All Ages* (Disabled Living Foundation, London)

Mandelstam, D. (1977) *Incontinence* (Heinemann Medical Books, for

the Disabled Living Foundation, London)
Montgomery, E. (1974) *Regaining Bladder Control* (Wright, Bristol)

Bibliography

Mandelstam, D. and Lane, P. (compilers) (1981) *Incontinence Bibliography* (Disabled Living Foundation, London)

GLOSSARY

Ano-rectal Agenesis: lack of complete and normal development in anus and rectum

Anus: excretory opening at the end of the bowel

Bacteriuria: presence of bacteria in the urine

Bladder: reservoir for urine

    Unstable Bladder: see Detrusor

Calculi (Urinary): stones formed in various parts of the urinary tract

Cystitis: inflammation of the bladder

Cystometry: a method of measuring pressure within the bladder

Cystometrogram: a recording of bladder pressure

Cystoscope: an instrument for viewing the inside of the bladder

Detrusor: muscular wall of the bladder which contracts to empty the bladder

    Unstable Detrusor: uncontrolled contraction of this muscle

Diazepam: a tranquilliser

Diuretic: an agent which increases urine flow

Diverticulitis: inflammation of sacs developing in the wall of the large intestine

Dysfunction: any disturbance of function of an organ

Dyspareunia: pain and difficulty during sexual intercourse

Dyspnoea: shortness of breath

Dysuria: pain on passing urine

Dyssynergia: faulty co-ordination of groups of organs and muscles

Electromyography: the study of electric currents in muscle fibres

Endoscopy: inspection of internal cavities of hollow organs

Enuresis: involuntary micturition

Faeces: waste matter from the bowel

    Impacted Faeces: large accumulation of faeces which is impossible to expel

Fistula: an abnormal opening between hollow organs or between a hollow organ and a skin surface

Frequency: passage of urine seven times or more per day, and more than twice per night

Glycosuria: presence of sugar in the urine

Haematuria: blood in the urine

Hirschsprung's Disease: a condition causing distension of the large bowel associated with constipation

Hyperplasia: enlargement of an organ resulting from an increased number of cells

Hypnotic: a drug which induces sleep

Hysterectomy: removal of the uterus

Hysterotomy: opening the uterus by surgical incision

Intravenous Pyelogram (IVP): see Urography

Megacolon: distension of large bowel

Micturition: the act of passing urine

Neoplasm: abnormal growth, a tumour

Nervous System:
>   Central: the section of the system which controls and co-ordinates voluntary action
>   Autonomic: the section which controls involuntary action

Neuropathy: non-inflammatory disease of peripheral nerves

Nitrazepam: hypnotic drug

Oestrogen: female hormone

Overflow Incontinence: leakage of urine from a fully distended bladder

Paraplegia: paralysis of the lower half of the body

Pelvic Floor: the muscular floor of the pelvis

Phimosis: abnormal tightness of penile foreskin

Polydipsia: excessive thirst

Polynocturia: Polyuria at night

Polyuria: production and passage of large quantities of urine

Post-micturition Dribble: dribbling of urine after bladder has apparently been emptied

Proctitis: inflammation of anus or rectum

Progesterone: female hormone

Prolapse: descent of organ or part, e.g. uterus, vagina or bladder due to weakening of supporting structures.

Prostate Gland: gland surrounding the bladder neck and urethra in men

Prostatic Hypertrophy: enlargement of this gland

Proteinuria: presence of protein in the urine

Pyelonephritis: infection involving secretory part of the kidney

Pyuria: pus in the urine

Rectum: lowermost part of the large bowel connecting with the anus

Reflex: an immediate involuntary response

Retention (of Urine): inability to pass urine

Stress Incontinence: involuntary loss of urine on exertion due solely to mechanical factors

Uraemia: a condition resulting from failure of the kidneys to excrete waste products

Urethra: canal along which urine passes from bladder to be excreted

Ureters: the tubes through which urine passes from kidneys to bladder

Urethritis: inflammation of the urethra

Urethrotomy: enlarging calibre of urethra by internal cutting

Urgency: an overwhelming desire to pass urine requiring immediate emptying of the bladder, usually accompanied by increased frequency

Urge Incontinence: involuntary loss of urine associated with a strong desire to void

Urinary Tract – Lower: composed of bladder and urethra which form a functional unit

Urinary Diversion: diverting the passage of urine to the surface of the skin, or into the bowel

Urodynamics: a study of function of the lower urinary tract by means of pressure-flow measurements

Urography: radiological examination of urinary tract, excretion urogram (IVP) being a record of this

NOTES ON CONTRIBUTORS

Janet P. Blannin, SRN, Continence Nurse Adviser, St Martins Hospital, Bath, Avon.

Elizabeth C. Clay, SRN, RCNT (ret'd), formerly Nursing Officer, Geriatric Education Programmes, Dudley Road Hospital, Birmingham.

Roger C.L. Feneley, FRCS, Consultant Urologist, Department of Urology, Ham Green Hospital, Bristol.

Dorothy A. Mandelstam, MCSP, DipSocSc, Incontinence Adviser, Disabled Living Foundation and Royal Free Hospital; Chairman, Association of Continence Advisors.

J.A. Muir Gray, MB, ChB, DPH, Community Physician, Oxfordshire Area Health Authority.

Michael F. Green, MA, MB, BCh, FRCP, Consultant Physician, Geriatric Department, King Edward VII Hospital, Guernsey, Channel Islands.

Sir Alan G. Parks, FRCS (dec'd), formerly Consultant Surgeon, St Mark's Hospital and The London Hospital; and Honorary Consultant in Colon and Rectal Surgery, The British Army.

Angela M. Shepherd, MRCOG, MCSP, Associate Specialist, Clinical Investigation Unit, Ham Green Hospital, Bristol.

G.S.C. Sowry, MD, FRCP (ret'd), formerly Consultant Physician, Edgware General Hospital, Middlesex.

Stuart L. Stanton, FRCS, MRCOG, Senior Lecturer and Honorary Consultant, Department of Obstetrics and Gynaecology, St George's Hospital, London; formerly Consultant Obstetrician and Gynaecologist, St Helier Hospital, Surrey; and Research Fellow, Institute of Urology, London.

Monnica Stewart, MB, BS, DObst, RCOG, Community Physician (Adult Health), Basingstoke & Northants Health Authority; formerly Senior Clinical Medical Officer (Adult Health), Newham Health District, City and East London Area Health Authority (Teaching); and Assistant Physician, Department of Geriatric Medicine, Edgware General Hospital, Middlesex.

Julia Taylor, BSc Econ, AIMSW, Principal Social Services Officer, Hertfordshire County Council.

Thelma Thomas, MRCP, Medical Research Council Scientific Staff, Epidemiology and Medical Care Unit, Northwick Park Hospital, Harrow, Middlesex.

Malcolm Keith Thompson, MRCGP, DObst, RCOG, General Practitioner, Croydon, Surrey.

R.K. Turner, BA, DipPsychol (London), PhD, District Psychologist, Leicestershire District Psychology Service, Towers Hospital, Leicester.

INDEX